Pharmacological Denervation and Glaucoma

Monographs in Ophthalmology 2

SPRINGER-SCIENCE+BUSINESS MEDIA, B.V.

Ph. F. J. HOYNG

Pharmacological Denervation and Glaucoma

*A Clinical Trial Report with Guanethidine and
Adrenaline in One Eye Drop*

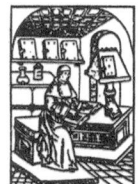

SPRINGER-SCIENCE+BUSINESS MEDIA, B.V.

Distributors:

for the United States and Canada
Kluwer Boston Inc.
190 Old Derby Street
Hingham, MA 02043
USA

for all other countries
Kluwer Academic Publishing Group
Distribution Center
P.O. Box 322
3300 AH Dordrecht
The Netherlands

Cover illustration
N^{+3} (stonehard)
Dutch tile, 16th century
Collection Gemeentemuseum, The Hague

ISBN 978-94-009-8676-3   ISBN 978-94-009-8674-9 (eBook)
DOI 10.1007/978-94-009-8674-9

Gelijkheid is een zaak van moeten. Ongelijkheid een van vrijheid.
Wie vrij is, is niet gelijk. Want, wij zijn niet gelijk.

J.H. van den Berg
In: *Leven in Meervoud*

Borné dans sa nature, infini dans ses voeux,
L'homme est un dieu tombé
qui se souvient des cieux.

Alphonse de Lamartine, 1790-1869
'L'Homme', in:
Premières meditations poétiques

Aan Marijke, Philippine en Jan Maarten

CONTENTS

Part two: *Clinical investigations*

INTRODUCTION

Glaucoma simplex or open angle glaucoma is a slow, progressive illness with an insidious course which can lead to blindness. According to our contemporary state of knowledge, the illness begins with a decreased outflow of aqueous humor. This leads, sometimes after a period of decreased aqueous humor production due to a feedback mechanism, to an increase in intraocular pressure (IOP). An elevated IOP can eventually lead to optic nerve damage, which manifests itself morphologically as glaucomatous papillary excavation and functionally in the development of a visual field defect. The classic triad of elevated IOP, papillary excavation and visual field defect, on which the diagnosis of glaucoma was also based in earlier times, is then present. To this can now only be added that tonography usually shows a decrease in aqueous humor outflow and that gonioscopy must reveal an open angle. On the basis of statistical findings, Goldmann has calculated that there may be an interval of as long as 18 years between the initial increase in IOP and the development of visual field defects. This point of view (which has been confirmed in practice) that the onset of the illness can be demonstrated by measurement of the IOP has introduced a new element into the discussion around glaucoma, namely, the concept of ocular hypertension. This implies simply that there is an (statistically) elevated intraocular pressure, even though the optic nerve may not (yet) be damaged.

It is not the purpose of this dissertation to enter into a discussion of theoretical explanations of the way in which damage to the optic nerve may arise; rather, I would like to limit myself to presenting a definition of glaucoma which has proven useful in practice, i.e. the loss of the equilibrium between the IOP and the capillary perfusion pressure in the vessels which supply the optic nerve. This definition leads to the concept of 'critical pressure', i.e. that IOP which does not actually damage the optic nerve. The diagnosis of 'glaucoma' can only be made retrospectively, when there is demonstrable damage. Knowing that an (statistically) elevated IOP can lead to optic nerve damage, it would be important to determine the critical pressure in an individual patient; unfortunately, this is not yet possible.

Since an elevated IOP can be present for a very long time before functional damage develops, one must take a large number of uncertain factors into consideration. For example, how high an intraocular pressure can the optic nerve tolerate and if a particular IOP is too high for the optic nerve, how long will it take before demonstrable damage develops? In other words, as long as there is no demonstrable damage, a patient with ocular hypertension is a glaucoma suspect. The term ocular hypertension should be considered to be synonymous with glaucoma suspect. This uncertainty is also reflected in the diversity of the percentages reported by various investigators with reference to the proportion of patients with ocular hypertension who will eventually develop functional changes, i.e. glaucoma.

What proportion of glaucoma suspects should be treated and at what IOP is one of the major problems in the conservative treatment of glaucoma. One fact is that the greater the deviation of the IOP from the (statistical) average, the smaller the chance that such an IOP is still normal. This has consequences for the criteria on the basis of which the decision to begin treatment is reached. One must also be aware of the fact that a decision to begin treatment of an elevated IOP implies that someone without complaints or subjective symptoms is turned into a patient receiving life-long therapy.

In addition to the level of the IOP and the duration of the elevation, a number of secondary factors such as age, family history, blood pressure, the condition of the blood vessels, the presence of diabetes mellitus and spontaneous platelet aggregration should also be taken into consideration in the decision whether or not to treat a case of ocular hypertension.

It is clear from the definition of glaucoma given above that we are dealing with two separate factors: the elevated IOP and the perfusion pressure in the capillaries which supply the optic nerve. The second factor is not measurable in man, but the first is. For this reason, the IOP is *the* parameter during the treatment of glaucoma, whether surgical or pharmacological. As such, the treatment of glaucoma is directed primarily at decreasing the intraocular pressure, which will result secondarily in better perfusion through the capillaries supplying the optic nervehead. Although our therapeutic arsenal has expanded over the years, miotic drugs have been the keystone of the pharmacological treatment of glaucoma for the past century. The principal objections against the miotic drugs are their side effects and their short duration of action, so that frequent application is necessary.

One substance which does not have the side effects of the miotic drugs and also does not have to be applied so often is adrenaline. Unfortunately, however, this substance by itself often has insufficient effect and in a very large proportion of the patients the necessary concentration (1-2%) eventually leads to manifestations of local allergy and intolerance, so that the treatment must be interrupted.

2

The stimulus for the present investigation was the availability of new combination consisting of adrenaline and guanethidine in one eyedrop, in concentrations which are lower than those in common use. The potentiating effect of guanethidine on the action of adrenaline can be expected to result in a greater effect on the intraocular pressure at a lower adrenaline concentration.

The purpose of this study was to investigate the effect of eyedrops containing guanethidine and adrenaline in combination in patients with open angle glaucoma and in glaucoma suspects, supplemental treatment being avoided as much as possible. The study extended over a period of 4 years (1976-1979) and involved 68 patients.

This dissertation divides naturally into two parts: the clinical investigation which we carried out is preceded by a pharmacological introduction dealing with the autonomic nervous system and the intraocular pressure, the concept of denervation and a review of the literature on the treatment of glaucoma patients by denervation, alone and in combination with adrenaline. This dissertation will be concluded by a review of the place of adrenergic therapy in the treatment of glaucoma and particularly the treatment with guanethidine and adrenaline in one eyedrop.

Ph. F.J. HOYNG

The Glaucoma Department of the
University Eye Clinic of Amsterdam
and The Netherlands Ophthalmic
Research Institute

3

PART ONE

PHARMACOLOGICAL INTRODUCTION

CHAPTER I

THE AUTONOMIC NERVOUS SYSTEM AND THE INTRAOCULAR PRESSURE

Introduction

The autonomic nervous system is responsible for the biological equilibrium in the body. Its activity is unvoluntary and falls outside the realm of consciousness. The autonomic nervous system can be divided into a sympathetic and parasympathetic part, which usually act antagonistically but sometimes synergistically in controlling the autonomic functions of the body. In 1934, Dale divided the autonomic nervous system up into a cholinergic and an adrenergic system, on the basis of the involvement of acetylcholine and noradrenaline, respectively. One of the functions of the autonomic nervous system is the regulation of the intraocular pressure. This is carried out partly by the sympathetic and partly by the parasympathetic system. An understanding of this regulatory process therefore requires an understanding of the anatomy, physiology and pharmacology of the sympathetic and parasympathetic innervation of the eye.

1.1 The sympathetic nervous system and the human eye

1.1.1 The anatomy of the sympathetic nervous system of the human eye

The sympathetic system which innervates the eye is composed of central, preganglionic and postganglionic nerve fibers. Inhibitory efferent fibers proceed from the center in the hypothalamus to the nucleus of Edinger-Westphal. In addition, efferent fibers proceed by way of the hypothalamicospinal tract (mostly crossed but also a few uncrossed) to the ciliospinal center of Budge, where they terminate in a synapse. Preganglionic myelinated fibers leave the ciliospinal center of Budge by way of the intermediolateral tract. Along the ventral roots of cervical nerve VIII and thoracic nerves I to III, sympathetic fibers leave the spinal cord in white communicating branches to form the cervical trunk. These fibers run through the inferior cervical ganglion via the medial ganglion to the superior cervical ganglion, where they have a synapse (Fig. 1).

Non-myelinated postganglionic fibers enter the skull by way of the carotid plexus and reach the eye via various pathways, i.e.:

a. fibers which proceed by way of Gasser's ganglion, the ophthalmic nerve and the nasociliary nerve and then split up into the long ciliary nerves, after which they enter the eye;

b. fibers which reach the interior of the eye by way of the ciliary ganglion and the short ciliary nerves.

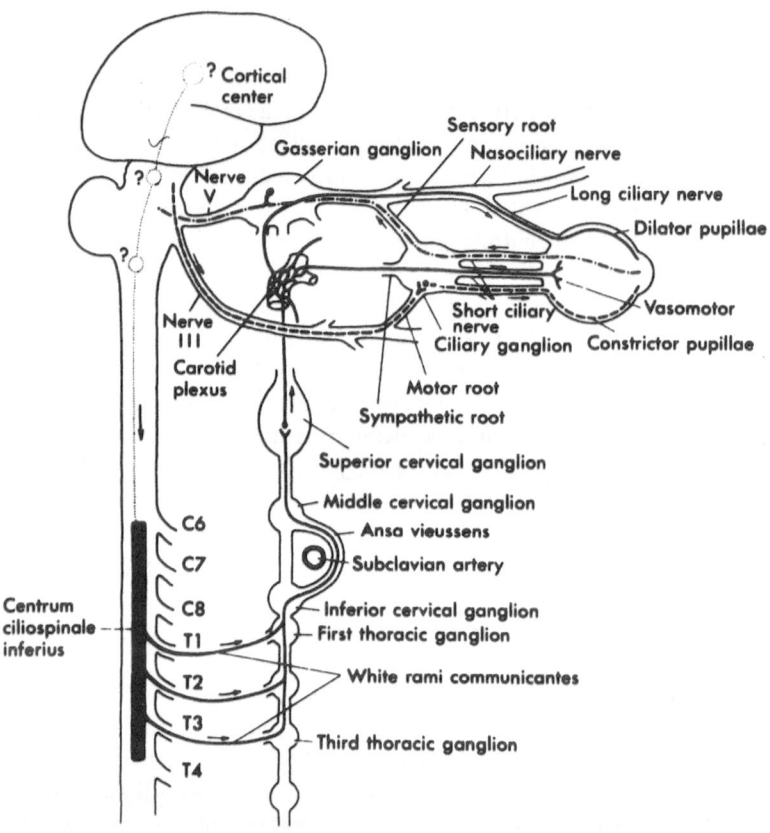

Fig. 1. The autonomic pathways to the eye (by courtesy of R. Moses, In Adler's: Physiology of the eye, p. 328, 1975).

1.1.2 The physiology of the sympathetic nervous system in the eye

The sympathetic fibers which reach the eye by way of the short ciliary nerves innervate the arteries, capillaries and veins of the intraocular tissues. Stimulation produces vasoconstriction and may decrease IOP. By way of the long ciliary nerves, the sympathetic fibers innervate the ciliary muscle and pupillary dilator. Stimulation of the sympathetic fibers innervating the dilator results in pupillary dilatation. Stimulation of the sympathetic fibers innervating the ciliary muscle results in relaxation of this muscle. Sympathetic fibers have also been described which innervate the chromatophores of the uvea; their function, however, is unclear.

1.1.3 The transfer of stimuli to the sympathetic receptor

The terminal organ of the sympathetic nervous system can be stimulated in two ways: by humoral transmission and neurohumoral transmission.

$$HO-\langle\rangle-CHOH-CH_2-HN-CH_3$$

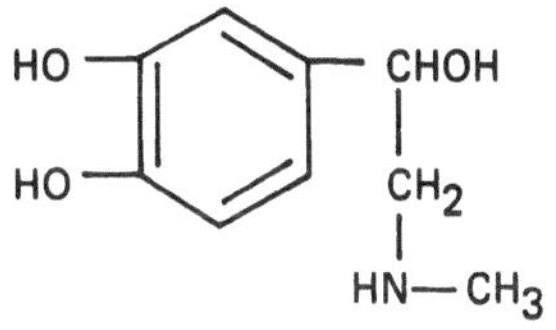

Fig. 2.   ADRENALINE

Humoral transmission is accomplished primarily by adrenaline (Fig. 2) and to a lesser extent by noradrenaline (Fig. 3). These catecholamines are synthesized in the adrenal medulla. Their secretion into the blood stream is controlled by the hypothalamus via the splanchnic nerve.

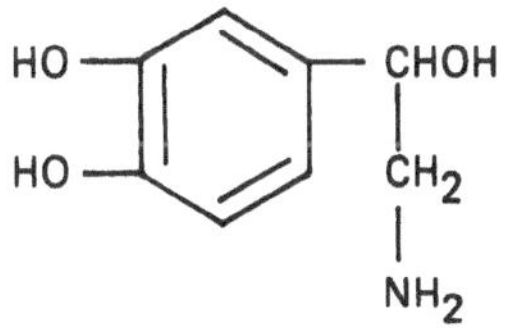

$$HO-\langle\rangle-CHOH-CH_2-NH_2$$

Fig. 3.   NORADRENALINE

In 1946, von Euler demonstrated that noradrenaline is the agent in sympathetic neurohumoral transmission. Noradrenaline is synthesized in the peripheral sympathetic neuron and stored in the granulated vesicles. These granulated vesicles reach the distal end of the nerve fiber by way of the axoplasmic stream. Excitation of the sympathetic neuron by an action potential (AP) results in depolarization and thus in a disturbance of the membrane potential of the axon. This results, in turn, in an increased permeability of the axon membrane leading to an influx of calcium ions in the axoplasm. Noradrenaline is then released from the granulated vesicles and from the axoplasm in the distal part of the axon (Fig. 4). This noradrenaline stimulates the adrenergic receptor via the synaptic cleft, after which 90% of the

9

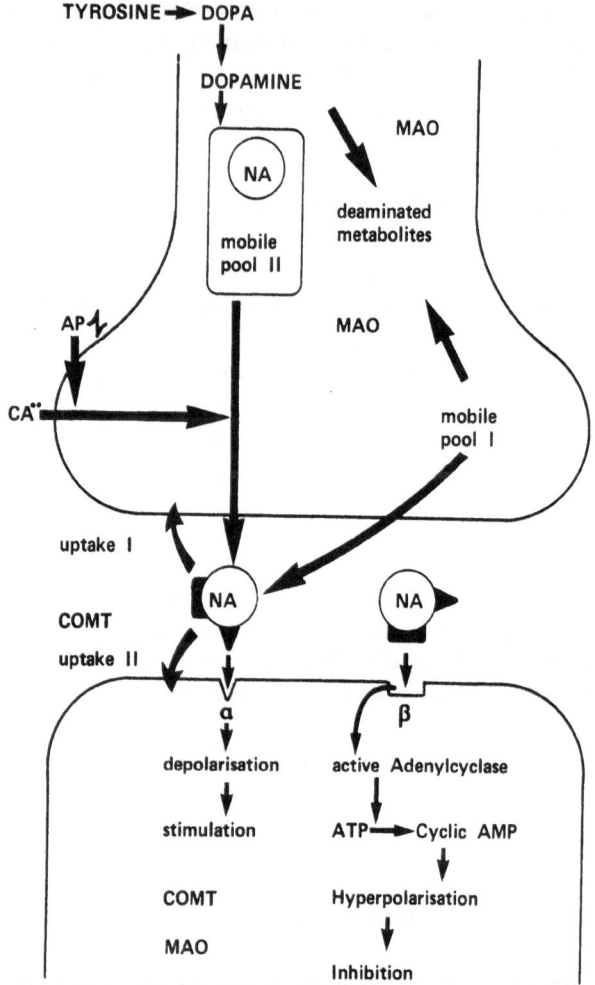

Fig. 4. Metabolism, release and effect of noradrenaline (NA) at the prejunctional, interjunctional and postjunctional site. For explanation and abbreviations see text (modified to Neufeld, 1979 and Goodman & Gilman, 1975).

noradrenaline is reabsorbed by the sympathetic nerve endings. In the neighborhood of the synaptic cleft (200-500 A), 5% of the free noradrenaline is deaminated by the enzyme monoamine-oxidase (MAO) in the mitochondria of the axoplasm of the nerve endings. Another 5% disappears into the circulation and is methylated by the enzyme catechol-O-methyltransferase (COMT). Both metabolites are further converted to 3-methoxy-4-hydroxy-mandelic acid (VMA).

1.1.4 The synthesis of adrenaline and noradrenaline

The synthesis of adrenaline of phenylalanine was suggested by Blaschko and Holtz as early as 1939. In 1947, Gurin and Delluva succeeded in demonstrating that radioactive adrenaline was produced in the adrenal medulla of rats after administration of radioactively labeled phenylalanine. Noradrenaline synthesis takes place in both the peripheral sympathetic neurons and the adrenal medulla, while adrenaline is only produced in the adrenal medulla.

The synthesis in the adrenal medulla proceeds as follows: the enzyme phenylalanine hydroxylase transforms the amino acid phenylalanine into tyrosine, which is then transformed into dihydroxy-phenylalanine (dopa) by the enzyme tyrosine hydroxylase. The transformation of dopa to dopamine is carried out by the enzyme dopa decarboxylase. Finally, dopamine is transformed into noradrenaline under the influence of dopamine-β-hydroxylase. Due to the presence of the enzyme phenylethanol N-methyltransferase, the adrenal medulla is able to transform noradrenaline into adrenaline. When the adrenal medulla is stimulated, it is primarily adrenaline which is liberated into the circulation, plus a very little noradrenaline (Fig. 5).

Tyrosine is taken up into the sympathetic neuron by means of an active transport mechanism and is than transformed into dopa in the mitochondria under the influence of the enzyme tyrosine hydroxylase. The dopa migrates into the cytoplasm, where it is transformed into dopamine by the enzyme dopa-decarboxylase. The dopamine is then concentrated in the granulated vesicles and transformed into noradrenaline by dopamine β-hydroxylase, after which the granulated vesicle with the noradrenaline leaves the perikaryon and migrates to the distal part of the axon by way of the axoplasmic stream. In the distal part of the axon, 95% of the noradrenaline is still stored in the granulated vesicles (mobile pool II) and only 5% is in free form (mobile pool I). (Fig. 4).

1.1.5 The adrenergic receptors

Whenever the sympathetic nervous system of the body is stimulated, then the sympathetically innervated organs and tissues react. The same adrenergic stimulus can, however, produce both stimulation and inhibition. As early as 1910, Barger and Dale noted that sympathomimetic amines have both an inhibitory and an excitatory action. They suggested the existence of two kinds of sympathetic receptors.

In 1948, Ahlquist classified the stimulatory and inhibitory effects of adrenaline and arrived at the postulate that there must be two kinds of adrenergic receptors, namely, α- and β-adrenergic receptors. Stimulation of the α-re-

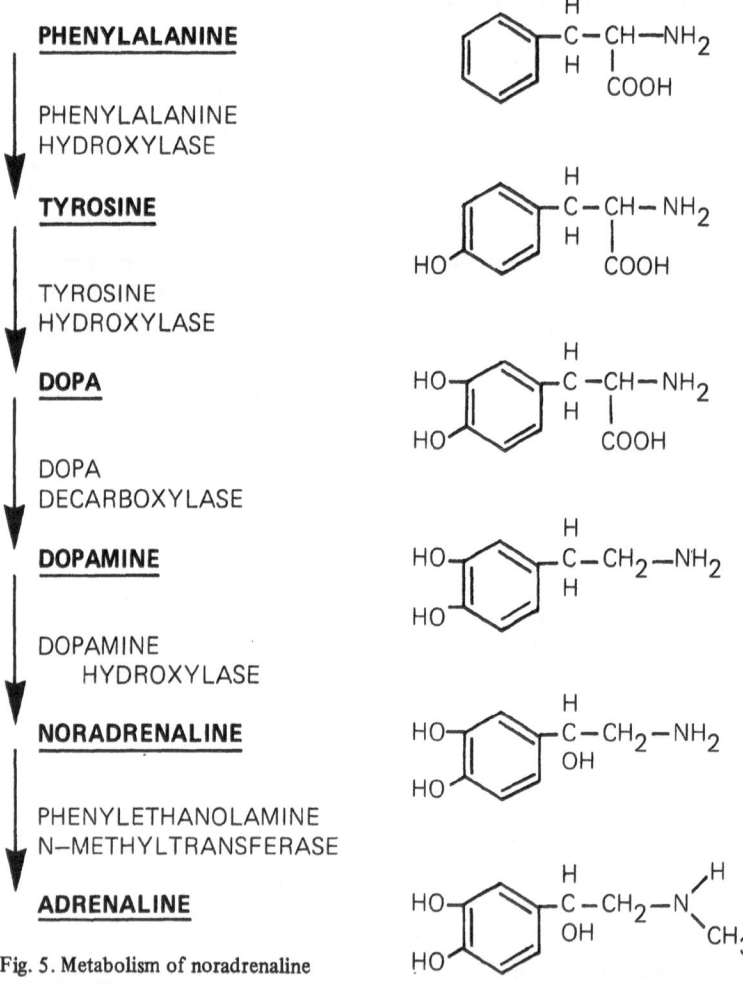

PHENYLALANINE

PHENYLALANINE
HYDROXYLASE

TYROSINE

TYROSINE
HYDROXYLASE

DOPA

DOPA
DECARBOXYLASE

DOPAMINE

DOPAMINE
HYDROXYLASE

NORADRENALINE

PHENYLETHANOLAMINE
N—METHYLTRANSFERASE

ADRENALINE

Fig. 5. Metabolism of noradrenaline and adrenaline.

ceptors would result in stimulation, while that of the β-receptors would cause inhibition. Later, Lands et al. (1967) divided the β-receptors into β_1 - and β_2 -receptors. The β_1 -receptors were said to exert a stimulatory effect on the action of the heart, while the β_2 -receptors were said to exert inhibitory effects on the blood vessel wall, the bronchial musculature and the motility of the intestines. In the eye, stimulation of the β_2 -receptors produce vasodilatation of the conjunctival blood vessels and a decrease in intraocular pressure due to inhibition of the production of aqueous humor. It induces relaxation of the ciliary muscle.

12

Recently, it has been demonstrated that there are probably also two kinds of α-adrenergic receptors. Langer (1974) and Wikberg (1978) have divided the α-receptors into α_1- and α_2-receptors, whereby the α_1-receptors are postsynaptic in localization, exert an alpha-stimulatory effect and show the highest affinity for phenylephrine, while the α_2-receptors are presynaptic, exert an inhibitory effect and show the highest affinity for clonidine. However, some authors have shown evidence of postjunctional localisation of α_2-receptors and presumable evidence of prejunctional localisation of α_1-receptors. (Timmermans et al., 1979; Drew et al., 1979; Starke et al., 1979; Docherty et al., 1979).

Receptors function at the molecular level. On the outer wall of the effector cell there are membrane-bound macromolecular functional units which are referred to as receptor sites. These sites combine with the transmitter to form a biologically active unit. After this combination has taken place, processes arise in the effector cell which lead to the α- or β-effect (Furchgott, 1960). Whether an α- or a β-effect is produced seems to be determined by the group on the transmitter molecule which is bound to the effector cell. In 1964, Ariens suggested that after administration of adrenaline, an α-adrenergic effect is produced by binding of the amino group to the effector cell, while a β-adrenergic effect is produced by binding of the catechol-hydroxyl group.

After binding of a particular molecular group of the biologically active transmitter to an α-receptor site on the outer wall of the receptorcell membrane, the enzyme ATP-ase is activated and a high-energy phosphate group is splitt off from ATP; this can result in depolarization of the effector cell and subsequently in contraction of smooth muscle cells. Binding to a β-receptor site is thought to lead to intracellular activation of the enzyme adenylcyclase, so that ATP is concerted to cyclic AMP (Fig. 4). E. W. Sutherland (1960) has called cyclic AMP 'the second messenger' of the adrenergic system. An increase in the level of cyclic AMP results in hyperpolarization of the effector cell and thus in relaxation of the smooth muscle cells, while a decrease in the level of cyclic AMP facilitates depolarization of the effector cell and thus contraction of the smooth muscle cells.

Sympathomimetic agents have either an α-adrenergic or a β-adrenergic action, or sometimes both. The sympathetic transmitter noradrenaline results primarily in α-receptor stimulation while the synthetic drug isoproterenol stimulates primarily the β_1-and β_2-receptors. Adrenaline seems to stimulate both α- and β-receptors. Adrenaline is a racemic mixture: the levorotatory isomer is approximately 20 times as active as the dextorotatory isomer.

1.2 The parasympathetic nervous system and the human eye

1.2.1 The anatomy of the parasympathetic nervous system of the human eye

The efferent preganglionic parasympathetic fibers which innervate the interior of the eye arise in the small cells of the nucleus of Edinger-Westphal. As part of the oculomotor nerve, these fibers proceed through the anterior part of the brain stem to the sinus cavernosus, from where they enter the orbit by way of the superior orbital fissure. In the orbit, part of the nerve branches off to innervate the inferior oblique muscle. This branch also contains the parasympathetic fibers for the eye, fibers which have either a synapse in the ciliary ganglion or one in the accessory ciliary ganglion of Von Axenfeldt. The postsynaptic fibers leaving the ciliary ganglion penetrate the sclera via the short ciliary nerves, while those proceeding from the episcleral accessory ganglion of Von Axenfeldt also penetrate the sclera and terminate in the eye (Fig. 1).

1.2.2 The physiology of the parasympathetic nervous system of the human eye

The parasympathetic fibers which reach the eye via the short ciliary nerves innervate the muscle of the pupillary sphincter and the ciliary muscle. Stimulation of the parasympathetic system via either the nucleus of Edinger-Westphal or the ciliary ganglion results in contraction of both the sphincter and the ciliary muscle. The accessory ciliary ganglion of Von Axenfeldt contains parasympathetic fibers which results in constriction of the pupil and the ciliary muscle in response to convergence stimulation. Acetylcholine is the neurohumoral transmitter for the preganglionic sympathetic, preganglionic parasympathetic and postganglionic parasympathetic fibers.

1.2.3 The parasympathetic receptor

In 1926, Loewi et al. discovered that acetylcholine is the 'vagus substance', i.e. the parasympathetic transmitter. Postganglionically, this substance is the neurohumoral stimulator of the parasympathetically innervated smooth musculature of the eye. An electrochemical stimulus results in liberation of acetylcholine from the ends of the axons and an increased membrane permeability on the side of the parasympathetic receptor, so that sodium ions enter and potassium ions leave the effector cell. This results in turn in depolarization. If the depolarization is sufficient, it is followed by an excitatory post-synaptic potential which produces contraction of the smooth muscle fiber. The acetylcholine which was liberated is deactivated by the enzyme cholinesterase.

1.3 The aqueous humor dynamics and the autonomic nervous system

1.3.1 Introduction

The autonomic nervous system keeps the intraocular pressure in balance by garanteeing homeostasis between the production and outflow of aqueous humor. The production of aqueous humor takes place in the ciliary body, while the outflow of aqueous humor runs by way of the trabecular network, the canal of Schlemm and the intra- en episcleral collector-veins.

A disturbance in the equilibrium between production and outflow of aqueous humor can result either in an elevated intraocular pressure, i.e. glaucoma, or in a decreased intraocular pressure which may lead to atrophy of the eye. The autonomic nervous system exerts its effect on the intraocular pressure by its innervation of the smooth musculature and the blood vessels, as well as possibly by way of an effect on the cells of the trabecular meshwork, the inner wall of the canal of Schlemm, and on epithelial cells of the ciliary processes. In a normal eye with a deep anterior chamber, pupillary constriction due to predominance of the sphincter muscle or pupillary dilatation due to predominance of the dilator muscle will produce no change in the course of the intraocular pressure.

Recently, in cynamolgus monkeys, Kaufman (1979) was able to show that after total iridectomy and intravenous administration of pilocarpine, the response of the iridectomized eye was identical to that of the unoperated control eye. He concluded that the iris plays essentially no role in the changes in intraocular pressure and outflow facility following pilocarpine.

On the other hand, contraction of the ciliary muscle as a result of cholinergic stimulation with, for example, pilocarpine produces a decrease in intraocular pressure due to a greater pull on the scleral spur. The fact that the trabecular meshwork is pulled open results in an increased outflow of aqueous humor. This was demonstrated in experiments on primates, (Kaufman and Barany 1976 and 1977). Desinsertion of the ciliary muscle at the scleral spur abolishes the increase in outflow facility normally produced by pilocarpine. It is not known whether relaxation of the ciliary muscle due to the β-adrenergic stimulation has any effect on the outflow resistance and thus on the intraocular pressure.

With the aid of isolated-muscle preparations of the sphincter and dilator muscles and the ciliary muscle, Van Alphen (1965, 1976), investigated the distribution of the α- and β-receptors in various species. He found that the dilator in man contains mainly α-receptors and very few β-receptors, while in the sphincter there are equal numbers of α- and β-receptors and the ciliary muscle contains mainly β-receptors with only a few α-receptors (Fig. 6).

	Dilator	*Sphincter*	*Ciliary muscle*
Cat	Mainly α, Some β	Mainly β, Some α	Mainly β, Some α
Rabbit	Mainly α, Few β	Mainly β, Few α	Mainly α, Few β
Monkey	Mainly α, Very few β	Mainly α, Perhaps β	Exclusively β, No α
Man	Mainly α Very few β	α and β in equal amounts	Mainly β Very few or no α

Fig. 6. Distribution of the adrenergic receptors in cat, rabbit, monkey and man (by courtesy of G.W.H.M. van Alphen, 1976).

In addition to the mechanical effect of the autonomic nervous system on intraocular pressure via the intraocular muscles, the autonomic nervous system also has an important effect on the not directly muscular structures in the eye. Here again, the distribution of the adrenergic receptors in the intraocular structures seems to vary from species to species. The distribution of α- and β-adrenergic receptors in the vascular bed and epithelium of the ciliary processes, the trabecular system, the canal of Schlemm and the intra- and episcleral collector-veins can only be studied by analyzing the responses to adrenergic stimulants and antagonists in the intact and perfused eye.

Since a human eye, pretreated with anticoagulant, is rarely available for perfusion, the study of the inflow and outflow of aqueous humor in man must rely on tonography, tonometry, measurement of the episcleral venous pressure and fluorometry, a technique introduced by Goldmann in 1951. There are a number of uncertain factors in tonography: for instance, the changes in episcleral venous pressure, and in corneal and scleral rigidity, the effect of the ipsilateral on the contralateral eye, the changes in 'pseudofacility' (representing 10-20% of the gross outflow in man, Bill 1977) and in uveoscleral outflow (up to 20% of the gross outflow in the elderly, Bill 1977). The episcleral venous pressure is usually assumed to be 10 mm Hg. Fluorometry is not frequently used for studies in man. Despite all this, an attempt will be made here to arrive at a working hypothesis for the human eye on basis of the results of various investigators. Whenever the results of studies in man are insufficient or unclear, these will be supplemented by data obtained from animal experiments.

1.3.2 The effect of adrenergic agents and antagonists on aqueous humor dynamics

The specific α-adrenergic agent is the neurohumoral transmitter noradrenaline. In 1971, Langham et al. observed a decrease in intraocular pressure in normal eyes after administration of 8.5% noradrenaline, accompanied by an improvement in outflow facility. In 1973, Gaasterland et al. reported that 2% noradrenaline produced no decrease in IOP in normal eyes, but did result in decrease in 'pseudofacility'. The episcleral venous pressure remained unchanged and instead of inhibition of aqueous humor production they reported an increase which was just below the level of significance. During treatment of glaucoma patients with 2,3% and 4% noradrenaline, Pollack (1973-1975) observed a decrease in IOP of about 20% and a 49% improvement in outflow facility. There was no demonstrable effect on the production of aqueous humor.

In summary, in both the normal human eye and the glaucomatous eye, α-adrenergic stimulation produces a decrease in intraocular pressure which is the result of an increase in outflow facility; there is no change in aqueous humor production.

The specific β-adrenergic agent is isoproterenol. In normal eyes, Langham et al. (1971) observed a decrease in IOP after isoproterenol which was accompanied by inhibition of aqueous humor production. In a later publication, Langham et al. (1974) also reported an increase in outflow facility. In 1973, however, Gaasterland et al. observed a decrease in IOP, inhibition of aqueous humor production and a decrease in 'gross facility' and 'pseudofacility' in normal eyes after isoproterenol. The episcleral venous pressure remained unchanged. As early as 1964, Bonomi had reported a 25% decrease being caused mainly by inhibition of aqueous humor production and to a lesser extent by an increase in outflow facility.

In glaucoma suspects treated with isoproterenol, Ross et al. (1970) observed a decrease in IOP which was due to inhibition of aqueous production; there was no demonstrable effect on the outflow of aqueous humor.

According to Langham et al. (1974), salbutamol, a powerfull β_2-adrenergic agent produces a decrease in IOP as a result of inhibition of aqueous production and an increase in outflow facility.

In summary, β-adrenergic stimulation produces a decrease in IOP in the human eye which can be ascribed primarily to inhibition of aqueous humor production and to a lesser extent to an increase in outflow facility. The role of the β-adrenergic receptor in mediating the outflow facility is unclear. Since Sutherland established cyclic AMP as the 'second messenger' of the adrenergic system in 1960, it has become possible to investigate the role of the membrane-bound β-receptor in relation to the outflow facility with the aid of this substance. After an injection of cyclic AMP into anterior chamber, Neufeld et al. observed an increase in outflow facility in both rabbits (1975a) and primates (1975b). Although these studies were not done in human eyes, his work suggests an active effect of β-receptor stimulation on outflow facility mediated by cyclic AMP (Neufeld 1973, 1978). The β-receptors are presumed to be located on the outer wall of the cell membranes of the endothelial part of the trabecular system and on the inner wall of the canal of Schlemm. At these sites, the outflow of aqueous humor meets the greatest resistance.

Adrenaline is a mixed adrenergic agent with a effect on both the α- and β-receptors. With the aid of fluorometry, Goldmann already showed in 1952 that application of adrenaline to the human eye resulted in inhibition of aqueous humor production. Kronfeld (1971) found that the initial inhibition of aqueous humor production was overlapped by an increase in outflow facility. After prolonged treatment of glaucoma patients with adrenaline, Becker (1958, 1961), Garner (1959) and Ballantine (1961) observed a gradual further increase in outflow facility. In normal eyes after application of 2% adrenaline, Gaasterland et al. (1973) observed a decrease in IOP with a decrease in both 'gross facility' and 'pseudofacility' and an inhibition of aqueous humor production. The episcleral venous pressure remained unchanged after adrenaline. Harris (1970) and Obstbaum (1974) reported an improvement in outflow facility after treatment of open-angle glaucoma patients and of glaucoma suspects, respectively, with adrenaline in concentrations of 1% or higher. With lower concentrations of adrenaline the decrease in ocular pressure was due to an inhibition of aqueous humor production. Recently, in normal human eyes, Townsend and Brubaker (1980) demonstrated an 18.6% increase in aqueous humor production after application of 1% adrenaline.

In summary, the decrease in ocular pressure produced by adrenaline at concentrations below 1% seems to be caused by adrenergic stimulation of the receptors which control the production of aqueous humor. At higher concentrations, the decrease in IOP is due to both, adrenergic stimulation of the receptors which control aqueous humor production and adrenergic stimulation of the receptors which control the outflow facility.

Finally, α-adrenergic blockade with 0.5% thymoxamine has no significant effect on intraocular pressure or outflow facility in either normal eyes or eyes with glaucoma (Wand 1976). Blockade with the $\beta_{1'2}$-receptor antagonist timolol maleate also has no effect on the outflow facility in the human eye (Zimmerman 1977; Sonntag et al. 1978, 1979).

1.3.3 The effect of parasympathetic stimulation on the ciliary processes and the intraocular pressure

The effect of acetylcholine and parasympathomimetic agents on the ciliary processes in the eye is unclear. It is well known that these compounds can produce conjunctival hyperaemia, hyperaemia of the iris and occasionally opalescence in the anterior chamber. Wilke (1974) observed conjunctival hyperaemia and an increase in IOP in the human eye after pilocarpine. The episcleral venous pressure was increased and the episcleral veins were dilated.

In perfused cat eyes which had been pretreated with physostigmine (eserine), Van Alphen et al. (1966) observed an immediate discharge of fluorescein from the ciliary body after application of acetylcholine. They concluded that this was probably the result of ultrafiltration, due to changes in the blood-aqueous barrier. In the cat, this effect of eserine-acetylcholine was abolished by atrophine, hexanethonium (a ganglionic blocking agent) and sympathomimetic agents.

In cat eyes which were perfused in vitro, Macri et al. (1975) observed an increase in both aqueous humor production and outflow after electrical stimulation of the parasympathetic ciliary ganglion. Since the increase in the production of aqueous humor was pressure related, they concluded that the underlying cause was ultrafiltration in the ciliary body.

In the perfused eyes of anesthetized rabbits, in which the intraocular pressure was held contant, Cole (1974) observed a discharge of fluorescein into the aqueous humor from behind the pupil after application of acetylcholine. By intravenous administration of carbon particles as a tracer, he was able to detect an increase in the endothelial permeability of the vessels of the ciliary processes. It was suggested that the blood-aqueous humor barrier may have been penetrated by a rupture of the 'tight junctions' in the non-pigmented epithelial cells of the ciliary processes.

In 1973, Alm et al. observed a doubling of the blood flow to the ciliary processes, the iris and the ciliary muscle in primates after administration of pilocarpine. They concluded that there was a dilatation of the vascular bed. Since these studies in various species were done in partly in perfused and isolated eyes with a constant intraocular pressure, any effect from the central nervous system and from changes in blood perssure (i.e. perfusion pressure) which might be induced by acetylcholine could be excluded. On the basis of these results it can be concluded that acetylcholine exerts an effect on the vascular bed in the eye and hence on the intraocular pressure.

In order to explain the effects of parasympathomimetic and sympathomimetic agents on the vascular bed in the ciliary processes, Macri (1978) suggested the following hypothesis: the ciliary processes function in the same way as the kidney glomerulus, i.e. aqueous humor production is a process of ultrafiltration and is regulated by the autonomic nervous system via an effect on the afferent and efferent vessels. Constriction of the efferent vessels on the choroidal side of the ciliary processes would lead to ultrafiltration

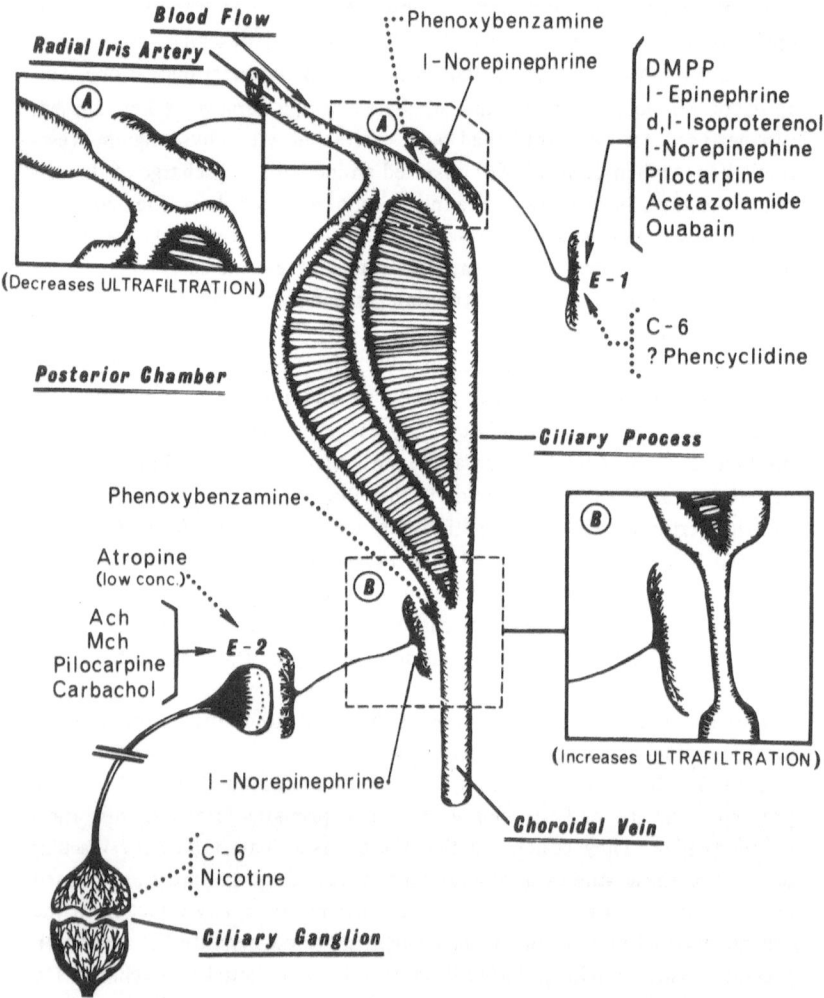

Fig. 7. Blood flow through the ciliary processes. Inflow by way of the radial iris artery and afferent capillaries, outflow by way of efferent capillaries to the choroidal venes. E1 and E2 are the hypothetical intermediary intraocular ganglions (by courtesy of F. Macri, 1978).

due to congestion of the vascular bed. Acetylcholine and other parasympathomimetic agents would produce such vasoconstriction by way of an intermediary intraocular ganglion (E2). Constriction of the afferent arterioles on the iridal side of the ciliary processes would lead to a decrease in the blood flow in the vascular bed, resulting in decreased ultrafiltration and aqueous humor production. This vasoconstriction would be produced by way of an intermediary intraocular synapse (E1), a synapse which is sensitive to sympathomimetic agents, diamox, ouabain and pilocarpine (Fig. 7). Although this hypothesis does not leave any room for a significant active role of the epithelium of the ciliary processes (Davson, 1969; Bito, 1977) and although the ganglia E1 and E2 have not been demonstrated anatomically, their existence is suggested by the blocking effect of hexamethonium (a ganglionic blocking agent) on the changes induced in the perfused eye by sympathomimetic and parasympathomimetic agents.

In summary, it seems very likely that the parasympathetic nervous system exerts an effect on the vessels of the ciliary processes via the ciliary ganglion. 'This opens the way for the participation of a central mechanism in the regulation of the intraocular pressure' (Macri, 1978).

CHAPTER II

THE PHARMACOLOGY OF THE EYE DURING
DENERVATION

2.1 Denervation, decentralization and supersensitivity

By 'denervation' is meant interruption of a nerve pathway at or behind
the last neuron. The interruption may be carried out surgically, such as
by ganglionectomy of the superior cervical ganglion, or pharmacologically.
When the nerve pathway is interrupted before the ganglion, one speaks
of 'decentralization'. Two weeks after denervation the effector cell develops increased sensitivity to directly acting agonists of the transmitter substances: noradrenaline for the sympathetic nervous system and acetylcholine for the parasympathetic nervous system. Indirectly acting agonists, in
contrast, have less or no effect on the effector cell after denervation (Burn
et al., 1931). The first phenomenon is called hyper- or supersensitivity while
the second is called subsensitivity. Agonists which exert their effect by re-
leasing the transmitter from the nerve endings are called indirectly acting
agonists and affect the effector cell via the last neuron; the directly acting
agonists act on the effector cell itself. Trendelenburg (1963) considers this
distinction between direct and indirect action to be too extreme and postu-
lates that the agonists of the transmitter substances fluctuate between these
two poles in their action.

Denervation of the sympathetic innervation of the eye is followed by development of Horner's syndrome (1889), consisting in man of ptosis and miosis and a fall in IOP.

The following discussion of the concepts denervation, decentralization and
supersensitivity is based on a review of the literature and will be limited as
much as possible to the eye.

*2.2 Paradoxical dilatation of the pupil and supersensitivity of the effector
cell after sympathetic and parasympathetic denervation*

Budge (1855) described an inexplicable dilatation of the pupil in the denervated eye after sympathectomy. In 1900, Langendorff called this reaction
'paradoxical dilatation of the pupil'. As early as 1880, Claude Bernard had
suggested that the sensitivity of tissues seems to increase when they are separated from the nerve fibers which dominate them.

After superior ganglionectomy in cats and rabbits, Meltzer and Auer (1904a, b) observed pupillary dilatation in the treated eyes after a small dose of adrenaline; the same dose of adrenaline had no effect on the normal contralateral eyes. A similar study was performed by Anderson (1904). He concluded that the denervated eye was supersensitive to adrenaline. Paradoxical dilatation of the pupil in the denervated eye was also noted in case of anxiety and excitation.

Elliot (1912) subjected cats to adrenalectomy and demonstrated that the paradoxical pupillary dilatation which normally developed in case of anxiety and excitation was abolished. These findings are in agreement with those of Innemee (1979) who observed an inexplicably dilated pupil in the unilaterally denervated eyes of cats under general anaesthesia with α-d-glucochloralose. In my opinion, a response of the denervated eye (which is supersensitive to catecholamines) to a discharge of adrenaline from the adrenals into the blood stream during the excitation phase of anaesthesia could be an explanation for this phenomenon.

Luco (1937) demonstrated that supersensitivity exists not only for α-adrenergic stimulation but also for β-adrenergic stimulation. He observed a stronger inhibitory effect in the uterine horn and intestine of rabbits after denervation and stimulation with adrenaline.

The concept of supersensitivity is also valid for the parasympathetic nervous system. Anderson (1905) observed a stronger response of the paralyzed pupillary sphincter to application of pilocarpine in the denervated eye after removal of the ciliary ganglion. Shen et al. (1936) treated normal and denervated eyes with increasing concentrations of acetylcholine, from 1% to 5%. In the parasympathetically denervated eyes there was a miotic reaction while the normal eyes did not respond. After pretreatment with physostigmine (eserine), an inhibitor of cholinesterase, a response was seen in the denervated eyes after as little as 0.01% acetylcholine. Due to the absence of the transmitter acetylcholine, no effect was seen in the parasympathetically denervated eyes with eserine alone. Recently, Colasanti (1979) observed a supersensitivity of the mechanisms which bring about a decrease in intraocular pressure in response to various concentrations of pilocarpine in rabbit eyes pretreated with mecholine.

In summary, supersensitivity for the directly acting agonists of the effector cell develops after either parasympathetic of sympathetic denervation.

2.3 Cross-over supersensitivity of both autonomic systems after denervation and Cannon's denervation law

By 'cross-over supersensitivity' is meant, for example, the development of supersensitivity in the effector not only for directly acting parasympathetic agonists, after denervation of the parasympathetic system, but also for sympathetic agonists and vice versa. Obviously, the effector organ must be innervated by both systems in such a case. In 1932, Rosenblueth observed not only supersensitivity to adrenaline but also to acetylcholine, pilocarpine and physostigmine after section of the sympathetic fibers innervating the nictitating membrane. When the parasympathetic system was blocked in cats by an intravenous injection of hexamethonium or pentolinium, Mantegazza (1958) observed a stronger response of the nictitating membrane and the capillaries to adrenaline. The cross-over supersensitivity was independent of both, the dosage administered and the duration of denervation.

However, recently, Colasanti et al. (1978) reported subsensitivity to cholinergic drugs in albino rabbit eyes after sympathetic denervation. It may be suggested that sympathetic decentralization, induced by intravenous hexamethonium and pentolinium by blocking the preganglionic sympathetic neurotransmission, is an explanation for the supersensitivity reported by Mantegazza. In any case, this supersensitivity is very similar to the supersensitivity reported after decentralization.

However, both normal supersensitivity and cross-over supersensitivity are subject to Cannon's law of denervation (1939). This law is reads as follows: 'When in a series of efferent neurons a unit is destroyed, an increased irritability to chemical agents develops in the isolated structures, the effect being maximal in the part directly denervated.' Emmelin (1961) feels that Cannon's law of denervation can justifiably be applied not only to surgical but also to pharmacological denervation and decentralization. This view is based on the fact, that both pharmacological and surgical decentralization produce less supersensitivity at the effector cell than pharmalogical and surgical denervation.

2.4 Supersensitivity and its relationship to the duration of sympathetic denervation

In 1935, Dale postulated that the store of transmitter in the nerve endings decreases when the nerve degenerates. The disappearance of the transmitter and the fact that it could no longer be liberated after denervation would then be the cause of the increased sensitivity of the denervated effector cell to chemical agonists. This postulate was based on the observation that there was hardly any supersensitivity in the effector cell immediately after denervation.

Also in 1935, Hampel followed the sensitivity of the nictitating membrane to adrenaline after superior cervical ganglionectomy and observed that the highly α-adrenergically innervated nictitating membrane showed an increasing sensitivity to adrenaline during the first 14 days. The maximum was reached at 14 days, after which the supersensitivity persisted for several months.

Various investigators have investigated the relationship between the disappearance of the transmitter and the development of supersensitivity in the effector cell. Burn and Rand (1959) found that the noradrenaline content in the iris of the cat was sharply reduced 11-17 days after either surgical or pharmacological denervation. They postulated a direct relationship between the degree of depletion of the transmitter and the degree of supersensitivity in the effector cell. Kirpekar et al. (1962) found, on the other hand, that the content of sympathetic amines in the nerve endings was unchanged after decentralization. Thus, decentralization was followed by supersensitivity in the absence of depletion (Trendelenburg et al., 1962).

Eakins and Eakins (1964) found that the noradrenaline content in the iris and ciliary processes of the rabbit approached zero 30 hours after cervical ganglionectomy. They also saw no difference in the noradrenaline content of the normal and denervated eye after preganglionic sympathectomy.

If a cat is treated with a large dose of intravenous reserpine, then stimulation via the superior cervical ganglion is blocked immediately but no demonstrable supersensitivity develops during the first few days (Fleming, 1961). If the treatment is repeated, the supersensitivity of the nictitating membrane to noradrenaline can be observed after 7 days, reaching a maximum after 28 days (Fleming, 1963). Fleming concluded that although the nerve stimulation is inhibited immediately after administration of reserpine, the development of supersensitivity requires more time. Supersensitivity does develop after a continuous very small dose of reserpine. This may indicate that the distal nerve endings do not have to be completely depleted before supersensitivity can develop in the effector cell. Trendelenburg (1963) suggested a direct relationship between the number of impulses which an effector cell normally receives and the speed with which supersensitivity develops after denervation. In addition to depletion of the transmitter from the denervated nerve endings there is a disturbance in the reabsorption of the transmitter by the nerve endings. In 1932, Burn postulated that the nerve endings of the adrenergic system may function as sites for the 're-uptake' (reabsorption) of sympathetic amines. When radioactively labelled noradrenaline was injected into the carotid artery of cats, the uptake was less in the denervated eye (Sears and Gillis, 1967; Kramer en Potts, 1969a). These investigators (Kramer and Potts, 1969b) showed that the amount of labelled noradrenaline taken up into the ciliary body of the denervated eye was inversely proportional to the degree of supersensitivity. Somewhat earlier, Kopin

(1968) had demonstrated a relationship between the decrease in noradrenaline uptake and chronic sympathetic denervation.

In summary, sympathetic denervation is followed by depletion of the transmitter noradrenaline, which is normally stored in the granulated vesicles, in the distal portion of the axon and by a block in the reabsorption of this transmitter, which normally amounts to 90% of the noradrenaline liberated. Both of these phenomena lead to supersensitivity of the adrenergic effector cell.

2.5 Denervation versus decentralization

It had already been pointed out earlier that the effects arising in the receptor cell after decentralization are not the same as those following denervation (Burn and Rand, 1959). The noradrenaline content in the iris of the cat is practically zero 14 days after denervation, while after decentralization it remains normal. Similar results were obtained by Eakins and Eakins (1964) in the rabbit iris and ciliary body.

Trendelenburg (1963, 1966) summarized the pharmacological differences as follows:

the supersensitivity induced by decentralization is relatively moderate and suspectible to the influence of directly and indirectly acting agonists of the transmitter. Decentralization does not result in depletion in the distal axons and the supersensitivity is independent of the degree of depletion;

the supersensitivity brought about by denervation is the result of a number of mutually interactive factors; these are the liberation of the transmitter, the block of its reabsorption and the depletion of the transmitter in the distal axon. Due to the absence of the transmitter, the effects of indirectly acting agonists are blocked. The supersensitivity resulting from denervation is many times more pronounced than that produced by decentralization. For this reason, decentralization is of no significance in the conservative treatment of glaucoma.

2.6 What is the cause of supersensitivity of the sympathetic receptor cell after denervation?

Up to the present, the fundamental cause of the development of supersensitivity after denervation remains unclear. The first theories which attempted to explain this supersensitivity sought the cause in a failure of the enzyme systems which catabolize noradrenaline. Denervation results in degeneration of the distal nerve endings (as demonstrated by Tranzer et al., 1968, with the aid of electron micrsocopy and 6-hydroxydopamine). The enzyme monoamine oxidase (MAO) is no longer able to break down the administered noradrenaline. This could be an explanation of the increased activity of the effector cell (Burn, 1952). The application of MAO-inhibitors should then result in supersensitivity to noradrenaline; this is, however, not the case (Balzer et al., 1956). In fact, pretreatment with the MAO-inhibitor tranylcypromine inhibits the decrease in intraocular pressure produced by noradrenaline in normal rabbit eyes (Hoyng and van Alphen, 1980).

COMT-inhibitors do not produce supersensitivity to either adrenaline or noradrenaline (Crout, 1961). Furthermore, Waltman and Sears (1964) reported an insignificant effect on COMT levels and a significant decrease (46%) in MAO content of the iris of albino rabbits after bilateral cervical ganglionectomy. It was concluded that it is unlikely that the supersensitivity following denervation is related to either a change in COMT activity or the moderate change in MAO activity.

Since 90% of the noradrenaline liberated is normally reabsorbed and the noradrenaline is eliminated from the synaptic cleft in this way, blocking of the re-uptake mechanism by denervation could well result in an increased and prolonged effect on the effector cell after noradrenaline application (Veldstra, 1956). The main objection to this theory is that it applies mainly to noradrenaline and is much less valid for the supersensitivity which can be demonstrated after adrenaline or isoproterenol. After all, the re-uptake mechanism seems most effective for noradrenaline. Blocking the liberation of noradrenaline from the granulated vesicles with the aid of bretylium results in only mild supersensitivity of the effector cell (Trendelenburg et al., 1962).

The most important factors playing a role in the development of supersensitivity are the liberation of noradrenaline, the depletion of the granulated vesicles in the distal axon and the block of the re-uptake mechnism. The more complete the depletion, the greater the supersensitivity (see above). However, this theory is also not water-tight.

It is a well known fact that the response of the effector cell to tyramine is reëstablished after prolonged denervation with reserpine and administration of small amounts or noradrenaline. Since tyramine acts indirectly by liberating noradrenaline from the distal axon, administration of noradrenaline or adrenaline must help to restore the functions of the axon after prolonged denervation. This may be the result of partial recovery of the re-uptake mechanism, reactivation of the synthesis of noradrenaline by the neuron, or partial restoration of the axon membrane potential. However, continued application of adrenaline in glaucoma patients who have been pharmacologically denervated with the guanethidine produces no decrease in supersensitivity. The longer the patients are treated with this combination, the greater the decrease in intraocular pressure and hence also the greater the supersensitivity to adrenaline. This shows that the theory of depletion and re-uptake in the distal axon as the cause of supersensitivity is also not water-tight.

Recently, Glaubiger et al. (1978) and Page et al. (1978) reported an increase in the density of the membrane-bound β-receptors after chronic denervation with guanethidine and 6-hydroxydopamine, respectively. No increase in the number of membrane-bound α-receptors could be demonstrated. A remarkable study is the one by Neufeld (1978) which demonstrated that the number of membrane-bound β-receptors decreased after treatment with adrenaline. With the electron microscope, Flach (1978, 1979) demonstrated degeneration of the distal part of the sympathetic axon in cats after supralethal doses of adrenaline. He also found a low noradrenaline content in the iris and spleen. This indicates that adrenaline by itself can produce a certain degree of denervation.

An increase in the number of β-receptors could explain the supersensitivity of the effector cell after denervation. However, this explanation would not be valid for the α-receptors. One possible explanation for the supersensitivity of the α-receptors is the following: Lanser (1974) and Wikberg (1978) described the pharmacological properties of the α_1- and α_2-receptors. The α_2-receptor is found primarily presynaptically, is supposed to exert an inhibitory effect and is maximally stimulated by clonidine, while the α_1-receptor is more often postsynaptic, is supposed to have a stimulatory α-adrenergic effect on the effector cell and is maximally activated by phenylephrine.

Hypothesis: When the distal axon degenerates during denervation, then the α_2-receptors, which are primarily presynaptic in localization, may lose their inhibitory effect on the effector cell. Due to this loss of their inhibitory activity, the postsynaptic effector cell may become hypersensitive to α-adrenergic stimulation; in other words, supersensitivity to directly acting α-adrenergic agonists may develop.

In summary, a disturbance in the axon membrane potential, an inhibition of the reabsorption of noradrenaline and a depletion of the noradrenaline stores in the granulated vesicles would seem to be the primary factors leading to supersensitivity of the effector cell and after denervation. As a result of these factors, there is an increase in the number of membrane-bound β-receptors in the effector cell and the α_2-receptors may lose their inhibitory effect on the effector cell due to depletion of noradrenaline in the distal portion of the axon and the synaptic cleft, so that supersensitivity to α-adrenergic stimulation develops.

2.7 Supersensitivity and the aqueous humor dynamics after denervation

Both electrical stimulation and section of the cervical sympathetic trunk result in a decrease in intraocular pressure, but the mechnisms producing this decrease are not the same. After electrical stimulation of preganglionic sympathetic fibers, the intraocular pressure in rabbits decreases by 25%. This decrease is caused by inhibition of aqueous humor production and not by an increase in outflow facility (Langham and Rosenthal, 1964, 1966).

Langham and Taylor (1959, 1960 a and b), who studied the changes in intraocular pressure and aqueous humor dynamics after pre- and postganglionic cervical sympathectomy in rabbits, observed no change in intraocular pressure immediately after the operation. Six hours later, a decrease in intraocular pressure appeared which reached a maximum 24-48 hours after the operation. Subsequently, the intraocular pressure gradually returned to normal. The fluorescein turnover rate was also determined after intravenous administration of fluorescein, and it was shown that the aqueous humor production was not affected by either denervation or decentralization. The authors concluded that the decrease in intraocular pressure immediately after denervation was caused by an increase in outflow facility.

Actually, this decrease is due to liberation of noradrenaline from the degenerating distal portion of the axon and is not yet due to supersensitivity of the effector; this develops only after 14 days (Sears and Barany, 1960). Prostaglandins which are produced after denervation may also play a role in the increase in outflow facility, presumably via cyclic AMP (Neufeld, 1973, 1975; Podos, 1973). The sensitivity to adrenaline of the mechanisms which regulate the outflow facility increase by a factor of 100-150 after denervation (Sears and Sherk, 1964; Eakins and Ryan, 1964). This reaction can be blocked by phenoxybenzamine, an α-receptor blocking agent, which indicates that the increase in outflow facility is due to supersensitivity of the α-adrenergic receptors (Sears and Barany, 1960; Eakins, 1963; Barany, 1962; Langham, 1966).

In 1964, Gnädinger and Barany observed an increase in outflow facility after isoproterenol in both denervated and normal rabbit eyes, but no supersensitivity to isoproterenol could be demonstrated in the denervated eyes. In 1963, Sears and Sherk observed supersensitivity of the outflow facility after cervical ganglionectomy only with low doses of isoproterenol intravitreously. With higher doses, there was no detectable difference in outflow facility between denervated and normal rabbit eyes. The fact that supersensitivity develops only after low doses of isoproterenol was confirmed by Barany and Gnädinger (1964).

In summary, following surgical postganglionic sympathectomy, the mechanisms which regulate the outflow facility develop supersensitivity primarily to α-adrenergic agonists and only to a lesser extent to β-adrenergic agonists.

CHAPTER III

THE TREATMENT OF GLAUCOMA WITH
DENERVATION ALONE

3.1 Cervical sympathectomy as a treatment for glaucoma

In 1869, Horner described a syndrome consisting of ptosis, miosis and decreased ocular pressure after injury to the cervical sympathetic trunk. This led Abadie (1897) to suggest treating glaucoma patients by resection of the superior cervical ganglion. Jonnescó, in 1889, was the first to perform this operation. For some time thereafter, this operation was the accepted treatment for glaucoma, but the results were disappointing because the decrease in IOP was only of short duration and the effect was variable (Elschnig, 1912; Linksz, 1931).

In 1953, Miller investigated the behaviour of the IOP after local blockade of the stellate ganglion with procaine in 30 glaucoma patients. In patients with open angle glaucoma he noted an increase in IOP immediately after the blockade, which was followed by a temporary decrease. In chronic congestive glaucoma there was a decrease in IOP, but there was also danger of angle closure. Denervation with locally applied procaine was thus of little use in the treatment of glaucoma patients.

In summary, there is no place for surgical denervation in the treatment of either open angle or chronic congestive glaucoma.

3.2 Pharmacological denervation alone
Introduction

Pharmacological sympathetic denervation and supersensitivity to catecholamines in the eyes can be brought about by various substances. The best known and most widely used are guanethidine sulfate and 6-hydroxydopamine (6-HD). Their pharmacological activity will be described in the following paragraphs.

Bretylium tosylate (Ornid), an oral antihypertensive agent which blocks the release of noradrenaline from the sympathetic nerve endings, is hardly ever used (Tregubova, 1967; Treister et al., 1970). Protryptiline, a tricyclic antidepressant which is a competative inhibitor of noradrenaline was applied locally in glaucoma patients by Kitazawa in 1972, but without any significant consequences for the conservative treatment of glaucoma. Another substance, α-methyldopa, an antihypertensive agent, is metabolized in the axon to α-methylnoradrenaline, a false transmitter which displaces noradrenaline from the storage depots in the sympathetic nerve endings. This may lead to supersensitivity to catecholamines. This drug is also of no use in the treatment of glaucoma.

The results of the studies with guanethidine and 6-HD will be discussed in detail in the following pages.

3.2.1 Guanethidine

3.2.1.1 Pharmacology

Guanethidine sulfate [2-(octahydro-1-azocinyl) ethylguanidine sulfate] is a highly ionized substance which is difficultly soluble in lipids (Fig. 8). Due to these properties, it penetrates the blood-aqueous barrier only with difficulty (Davson, 1962). It is a postganglionic adrenergic neuron blocker, i.e. it blocks the response to sympathetic stimulation of the nerve. The α- and β-adrenergic responses are depressed to the same extent after guanethidine. After pretreatment with guanethidine, the response to indirect sympathomimetic agents such as tyramine and hydroxyamphetamine is reduced or completely abolished. This is the result of a decrease in the amount of noradrenaline which can be released after stimulation. Guanethidine produces depletion of noradrenaline in the sympathetic nerve endings. The symptoms which appear after prolonged treatment with guanethidine are identical to those after postganglionic denervation (Trendelenburg, 1963). This supports the opinion of Emmelin (1961) that the 'Law of Denervation' need not be limited to surgical denervation but is equally valid for pharmalogical denervation.

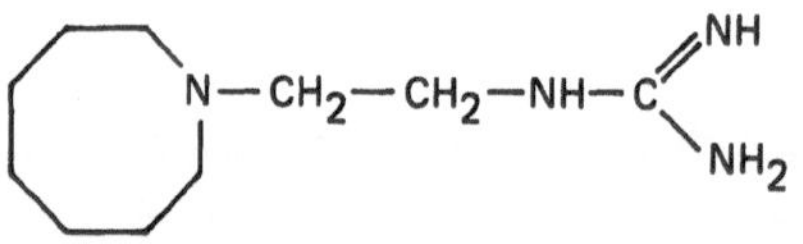

Fig. 8.   **GUANETHIDINE**

Supersensitivity of the sympathetic effector cell to directly acting sympathomimetic agents after pretreatment with guanethidine has been reported by various authors (Maxwell et al., 1960, a, b; Vernikos et al., 1960). In 1962, Boura and Green observed a maximal development of supersensitivity in the effector cell after 14 days' pretreatment with guanethidine. They found that the effect of noradrenaline was increased 50-100 fold while that of adrenaline was increased 20 fold.

Mitchell and Oates (1970) found that guanethidine is taken up into the sympathetic axon by the same membrane transport system as noradrenaline. When the membrane permeability is increased, noradrenaline is released. The reabsorption of the liberated noradrenaline is competitively inhibited by guanethidine, resulting in depletion of noradrenaline in the distal axon and consequent supersensitivity of the effector cell to directly acting sympathomimetic agents.

In 1964, Richardson demonstrated that the axons in which small granulated vesicles could be seen were adrenergic. In rabbits pretreated with intravitreous guanethidine, Tamura (1973) observed, with the aid of electron microscopy, a decrease in the number of small granulated vesicles and information of vacuoles in the distal portion of the sympathetic axon. These phenomena were reversible. The catecholamine fluorescence of the sympathetic fibers was also decreased after guanethidine, indicating a decrease in the content of noradrenaline in the sympathetic axons (Csillik, 1964; Tamura, 1973).

3.2.1.2 Guanethidine and the intraocular pressure in experimental animals: the rabbit eye

After damage to the corneal epithelium and application of guanethidine eyedrops, Oosterhuis (1962) noted a decrease in IOP and, after transitory mydriasis, miosis. When the cornea was left undamaged, then guanethidine concentrations increasing from 1% to 10% failed to produce a decrease in IOP.

In 1965, Hendley and Eakins investigated the aqueous humor dynamics, the course of the IOP and the catecholamine content in the iris and ciliary processes in rabbits. After a subcutaneous injection of guanethidine (20 mg/kg) they observed a decrease in IOP without any increase in outflow facility. Intravitreous injection of 100-200 mg of guanethidine, however, produced both a decrease in IOP and an increase in outflow facility. This difference in effect was explained on the basis of the poor penetration of guanethidine through the blood-aqueous barrier and not by the method of administration as such. In the same investigation, they found hardly any difference in the degree of depletion of noradrenaline in the iris and ciliary body 3 and 6 hours after subcutaneous or intravitreous administration of guanethidine. The only difference was that there was complete depletion of noradrenaline in the iris and ciliary body 24 hours after intravitreous administration compared to 70% depletion after subcutaneous injection.

The fact that the noradrenaline depletion is approximately the same after either subcutaneous or intravitreous administration does not indicate that the blood-aqueous barrier plays a significant role in preventing an increase in outflow facility after subcutaneous injection of guanethidine. After all, local intravitreous administration of guanethidine produces an immediate outpouring of noradrenaline from the sympathetic nerve endings in the iris and ciliary body, resulting in a relatively high noradrenaline concentration in the aqueous humor. This results in an increase in the outflow facility. A subcutaneous injection, on the other hand, releases a gradual low dosage of guanethidine which reaches the eye via the circulation and the blood-aqueous barrier. Although the degree of depletion is about the same in both cases, the release of noradrenaline is more uniform after subcutaneous injection. This therefore results in a lower noradrenaline concentration in the aqueous humor, so that there also can be no increase in outflow facility.

The course of the IOP after guanethidine and adrenaline, alone and in combination, was investigated by Lamble in 1973. After a single application of 5% guanethidine in eyedrops, there was a decrease in IOP in both the treated and contralateral untreated eye. The decrease in IOP after 0.25% adrenaline was more marked in both eyes when one eye of reach rabbit had been treated with guanethidine for one week than when they were treated with 0.25% adrenaline alone. After 3 weeks of continued treatment with 5% guanethidine and 0.25% adrenaline, tachyphylaxis developed in the effect on the IOP.

The effect of guanethidine on the IOP is not very impressive in rabbits compared to that in man. First we will discuss the effect of guanethidine alone on the human eye and the IOP in man, and then in a separate chapter we will discuss its combination with adrenaline.

3.2.1.3 Guanethidine in the human eye

A decrease in IOP after guanethidine was first reported by Keates et al. (1960). In 20 normal experimental subjects, a decrease in IOP of 2-4 mm Hg was observed after an intravenous injection of guanethidine. The maximal effect was reached 3 hours after administration. No ptosis or conjunctival hyperaemia were noted, althought in a few cases there was miosis. A remarkable decrease in IOP was observed in patients with primary open angle glaucoma.

In 1961, Küchle administered 10% guanethidine in eyedrops 3 times a day to glaucoma patients and normal controls. In both groups there was a marked decrease in IOP which was comparable to that after 1% pilocarpine. No effect on the outflow facility could be demonstrated.

A similar study was carried out by Kutschera in 1961. He found that in glaucoma patients, application of 10% guanethidine in eyedrops was followed by a 22% decrease in IOP lasting 12 hours. Side effects noted included mild ptosis, miosis and conjunctival hyperaemia. The decrease in IOP due to result of an increase in outflow facility and not due to inhibition of aqueous humor production. Stepanik (1961) also observed a decrease in IOP due to an increase in outflow facility glaucoma patients after a single application of 10% guanethidine.

In glaucoma patients who were insufficiently regulated on maximal therapy, Oosterhuis (1962) observed a decrease in IOP after addition of 10% guanethidine 1-3 times a day. He points out that the hyperaemia following guanethidine should not be locked upon as an effect of irritation but rather as a pure or direct vasodilatation. Although he also noted mild ptosis, he considered the treatment with guanethidine to be acceptable 'and calling for extensive investigation'.

Castren et al. (1962, 1968) treated glaucoma patients with 5% guanethidine 3 times a day and found that the decrease in IOP was due to a 50% inhibition of aqueous humor production. After a single application of guanethidine, the decrease in IOP reached a maximum of 37% in 7 hours. Dilation of the pupils was seen in a few cases during the first few hours after treatment, but after 2.5 hours most of the patients showed miosis. The miotic pupil reacted to light. In their study, 5% guanethidine had no effect on accomodation or the degree of opening the eyelid. However, during treatment with 10% guanethidine they noted a mild ptosis (1-2 mm).

Bonomi et al. (1967) also found that the decrease in IOP in normal and glaucomatous eyes after a single application of 10% guanethidine could be ascribed primarily to inhibition of aqueous humor production. A significant but transitory increase in outflow facility, 4 hours after application, was observed only in normal eyes. Since this biphasic effect on the aqueous humor dynamics corresponded to the biphasic action of topical noradrenaline, the authors concluded correctly that this phenomenon was caused by displacement of noradrenaline from the sympathetic nerve endings by guanethidine.

In 1967, Merté et al. used 10% guanethidine to treat patients with open angle glaucoma in whom the IOP decreased insufficiently on parasympathomimetic agents and concluded that patients with IOP lower than 30 mm Hg in the absence of therapy responded well to guanethidine. The effect of treatment could only be evaluated after at least 4 days. In this study there was again no effect on the outflow facility. Occasionally they noted a troublesome conjunctival hyperaemia which sometimes led to interruption of treatment.

Another way of investigating the aqueous humor dynamics is by means of fluorescein photometry. Both Anselmi et al. (1968) and Wolff (1969) demonstrated a decrease in the fluorescein turn-over rate in normal eyes after application of 10% guanethidine in eyedrops. This indicates inhibition of aqueous humor production.

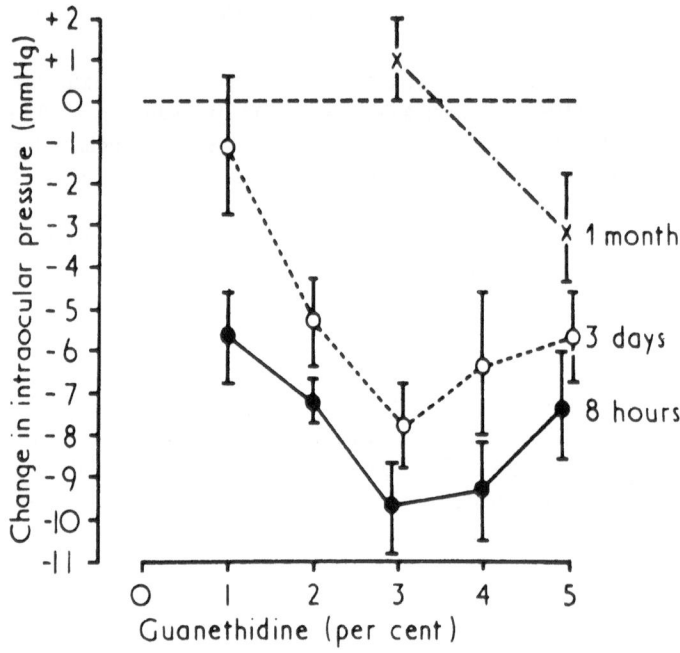

Fig. 9. Decrease in intraocular pressure in mm Hg during treatment with guanethidine 1-5% of 9 glaucoma suspects after 8 hrs, 3 days and 1 month (by courtesy of Paterson and Paterson, 1972).

Finally, I would like to mention the pioneering study of Paterson and Paterson (1972, 1974) in which they reported on 9 patients with ocular hypertension who were treated with increasing concentrations of guanethidine (from 1% to 5% twice a day). After a single application, they observed a decrease in IOP of 9.7 mm Hg with 3% guanethidine and 7.3 mm Hg with 5% guanethidine (Fig. 9). However, after one month of treatment, the decrease in IOP observed with 3% guanethidine alone had disappeared and the pressure was even 1 mm Hg higher than before the beginning of the treatment. With 5% guanethidine the IOP was still 3.2 mm Hg below the starting level. They explained this on basis of the absence of endogenous stores of noradrenaline in the sympathetic nerve endings as a result of depletion. After a single

36

application of 1-5% guanethidine there was an increase in outflow facility which reached a maximum at concentrations of 3% and higher. The measurements were carried out 4 hours after application.

In summary, application of guanethidine alone results in a fall in IOP but the effect diminishes when the treatment is continued. In patients with POAG the decrease in IOP is due to inhibition of aqueous humor production, while in normal eyes and eyes of glaucoma suspects an increase in outflow facility may also play a role. The opinions of the various investigators regarding the effect of guanethidine on the aqueous humor dynamics are divided.

3.2.2 6-Hydroxydopamine (6-HD)

3.2.2.1 Pharmacology

6-Hydroxydopamine (2, 4, 5-trihydroxyphenylethylamine) is an isomer of noradrenaline (Fig. 10). Due to its marked similarity to noradrenaline, 6-HD is readily taken up into the sympathetic nerve endings, so that the stored noradrenaline is released. The binding of 6-HD in the nerve ending is practically irreversible. resulting in a selective pharmacological denervation and degeneration in the distal sympathetic nerve ending. 6-HD is deactivated by oxidation.

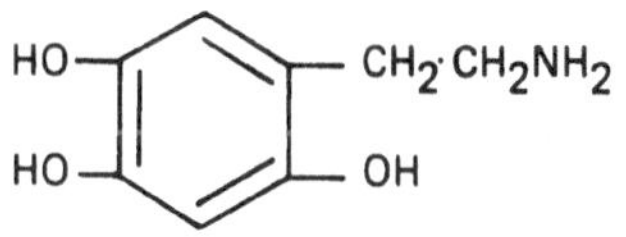

Fig. 10.   6 – HYDROXYDOPAMINE

Porter et al. (1962) reported a decrease in the catecholamine content of mouse heart after pretreatment with 6-HD. With the aid of electron microscopy, Tranzer and Thoenen (1968) observed acute degeneration of the adrenergic nerve endings of the iris, among other organs, in cats 3 days after an intraperitoneal injection of 6-HD. This degeneration was selective, i.e. cholinergic nerve endings were normal in appearance. In various organs the noradrenaline content decreased to less than 10% of normal. Two weeks after the treatment the sympathetic nerve endings had regained their normal form, but the granulated vesicles in the distal axons only reappeared 4 months after the treatment, indicating a prolonged depletion of noradrenaline. This selective degeneration could only be demonstrated in the distal

37

portion of the sympathetic axon and not in the perikaryon. The denervation process lasted 4 months and was reversible.

3.2.2.2 6-Hydroxydopamine in experimental animals

The effect of chemical denervation on the IOP, outflow facility and episcleral venous pressure was studied in owl monkeys and rabbits by Holland and Mims (1971). In owl monkeys they observed a 25-30% decrease in IOP one week after application of eyedrops containing 10% 6-HD. During the first week after denervation the outflow facility increased by 33%, but during the second week an increase in outflow facility could no longer be demonstrated. In rabbits there was only a transitory decrease in IOP and no significant supersensitivity to noradrenaline or isoproterenol. The episcleral venous pressure was also unchanged. In 1973, Kitazawa et al. investigated the best technique for the application and penetration of 6-HD (which is rather unstable) in rabbits. The greatest penetration of 6-HD was achieved by means of iontophoresis.

There is a difference in the mode of action of guanethidine and 6-HD. While denervation with 6-HD involves both degeneration and depletion of the distal sympathetic nerve endings, denervation with guanethidine results only in depletion of the noradrenaline stores, without degeneration (Csillik, 1964; Tamura, 1973).

CHAPTER IV

THE TREATMENT OF GLAUCOMA WITH
PHARMACOLOGICAL DENERVATION AND ADRENALINE

Introduction

Studies in patients with Horner's syndrome form the basis for the use of pharmacological denervation and adrenaline in the treatment of glaucoma. Horner himself (1869) had reported that the IOP was lower in patients with the syndrome which he had described. In 1920, Cobb et al. reported that the IOP was 5 mm Hg lower in patients with unilateral Horner's syndrome. The behaviour of the IOP and the aqueous humor dynamics were investigated in detail in one patient with unilateral Horner's syndrome by Swegmark (1963). The IOP on the affected side showed an average decrease of 3.7 mm Hg, which could be ascribed to decreased aqueous humor production.

On the basis of results obtained in denervated rabbit eyes which were treated with adrenaline (Sears, 1963; Eakins, 1964), Sears (1966) treated 19 patients with Horner's syndrome with topical 2% adrenaline. He noted that the mechanisms controlling the outflow facility were supersensitive to adrenaline.

In one patient with a clinical Horner's syndrome and one patient in whom a Horner's syndrome had been induced by guanethidine, Bron (1969) investigated the aqueous humor dynamics before and after local application of noradrenaline and adrenaline. In both affected eyes there was a decreased aqueous humor production compared to the contralateral normal eye. A single application of either noradrenaline or adrenaline was followed by an increase in aqueous humor production.

The research on glaucoma patients treated with pharmacological denervation can be divided into studies using guanethidine and those using 6-HD as an adrenergic blocking agent.

4.1 Guanethidine and adrenaline

4.1.1 Treatment with 5-10% guanethidine and 0.5-2% adrenaline, each applied separately

As early as 1966, Drance reported on the treatment of glaucoma patients with 10% guanethidine and 1% adrenaline. Although he observed no potentation of the effect on IOP in this pilot study, Drance suggested the use of this combination.

The study of 9 patients with ocular hypertension by G. Paterson and G.D. Paterson (1972, 1974) was of decisive importance. During treatment with guanethidine alone in concentration of 1-5%, the 3% solution was found to have become completely ineffective in lowering the IOP after one month of treatment, while the 5% solution still produced only a slight drop in IOP. In one patient, the outflow facility was measured 4 hours after the application of varying concentrations of guanethidine. With solutions of 3, 4 and 5% guanethidine, there was an increase in outflow facility by about 0.10 μl/mm ˉIg/min.

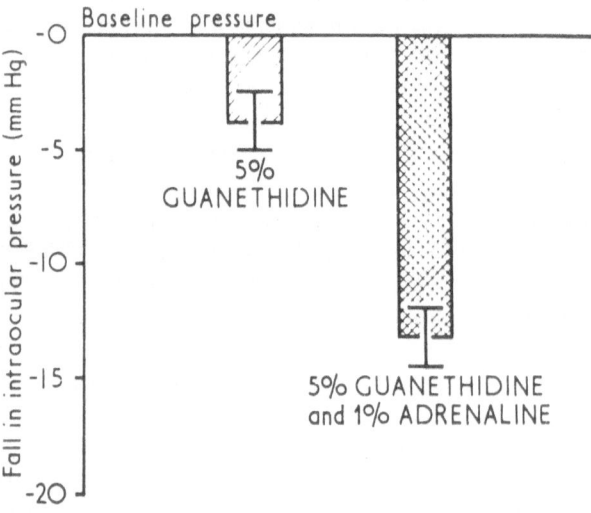

Fig. 11. Effect on intraocular pressure of adding 1% of adrenaline to guanethidine pretreated patients (by courtesy of Paterson and Paterson, 1972).

Since it turned out that the decrease in IOP produced by guanethidine alone could not be maintained, the investigators decided to try a combination of 5% guanethidine and 1% adrenaline. Now, after one month of treatment, the decrease in IOP averaged 13 mm Hg and increased further as the treatment was continued. The effect of 1% adrenaline alone on the IOP (a decrease of about 4.8 mm Hg, Becker and Ley, 1958) was thus potentiated.

In 1973, Roth treated 49 eyes in 29 glaucoma patients in whom maximal therapy was incompletely effective in regulating the IOP by addition of 5% guanethidine in combination with 0.25% or 0.5% adrenaline to the existing regimen. After a period of 11 months, approximately 50% of the original group was still under treatment with this combination, while in 16 eyes the IOP had become too high and in 4 eyes there had been troublesome side effects. Although the treatment was successful in only 50% of the patients, Roth pointed out that this was achieved in patients who would otherwise have had to undergo surgery.

A similar study was carried out by Gloster (1974). During 2.5-3 years, 42 glaucoma patients in whom previous therapy had been insufficiently effective were treated with 5% guanethidine. This produced an additional drop in IOP of 3 mm Hg, which was not increased further by simultaneous application of adrenaline. During the treatment, 13 patients had to be withdrawn from the study because IOP was not regulated and in 12 patients the treatment was interrupted because the side effects were too severe. Only one third of this group of patients was treated successfully. It is striking that the addition of adrenaline failed to produce a greater drop in IOP in this study.

Better results were obtained by Crombi (1974). After all previous therapy had been stopped, 35 eyes in 21 glaucoma patients who could not be brought under control by the use of drugs, were treated with 5% guanethidine and 1% adrenaline twice daily. Using this combination, the IOP was under control in 50% of the eyes after 2 years of treatment and in 43% after 3 years. The decrease in IOP was greater (10.5 mm Hg) when a combination of guanethidine and adrenaline was administered than with guanethidine alone (5.5 mm Hg). Conjunctival hyperaemia was noted in many patients but this did not always lead to cessation of treatment.

In 1974, Paterson et al. reported on their experiences over the past 4 years with 5% guanethidine and 1% adrenaline. During this period they treated 104 eyes in 56 glaucoma patients with this combination twice daily. Only 13 eyes were well regulated during the entire 4 years. In another 13 eyes a troublesome allergy developed consisting of swollen eyelids, conjunctival hyperaemia and punctate keratitis. Now and then mydriasis was seen during the first few hours after application. There was rarely ptosis, but a mild punctate keratitis was seen in one third of all cases. In 17 eyes, the adrenaline concentration was successfully reduced from 1% to 0.5%. The average decrease in IOP was 14-15 mm Hg. The younger the patient and the higher the IOP initially, the greater was the decrease in IOP. Despite the side effects, they considered the non-miotic therapy with guanethidine and adrenaline to be effective and suggested that the concentrations of the solutions should be reduced.

Etienne (1973) investigated the effects of 5% guanethidine twice daily and 2% adrenaline three times a day in 56 eyes of 35 glaucoma patients. Two weeks before the beginning of this study, all previous therapy was withdrawn. After control measurements in the absence of treatment, measurements were made during therapy 2 and 4 hours after each application. In 70% of the eyes the ocular pressure was decreased to values below 22 mm Hg. The average drop in IOP was 11.5 mm Hg after 3 months and 11.9 mm Hg after 6 months. In a few patients an IOP curve was recorded by the method of Harms (measurements every half hour for 4 hours after application). After a single application of either adrenaline alone or the combination of adrenaline and guanethidine, there was an initial drop in ocular pressure during the first hour, followed by a slight increase during the 2nd and 3rd hour after application. After 4 hours the IOP remained more of less constant. For this reason, Etienne suggests that the IOP should be evaluated about 3-4 hours after application of a drug. Patients who responded poorly to the combination were found to become resistant after 2 or 3 months. Patients with high IOP values in the absence of therapy who still showed values in the neighbourhood of 30 mm Hg during the first month despite a satisfactory fall in IOP often had an IOP below 22 mm Hg after 3 months of treatment. In 30% of the patients the IOP decreased further after a half year of treatment, while in 63% the drop in IOP was maximal after 2 months and was no greater after one year. In 7% the treatment had to be discontinued due to a not regulated IOP, allergy, ptosis or intolerance. Approximately 30% of the patients had conjunctival hyperaemia.

Jones et al. (1977) treated 35 patients with primary open angle glaucoma exclusively with 5% guanethidine and 1% adrenaline. During the first 6 months 9 patients had to be withdrawn from the study due to insufficient effect on the IOP and 6 patients withdrew because of troublesome side effects. After one year these figures had increased to 10 and 10, respectively, and after 3 years to 16 and 12. As a result, after 3 years of treatment only 7 patients remained who could be adequately regulated by means of this combination. The most troublesome side effects were conjunctival hyperaemia in an early stage and epiphora with rhinorrhoea in a later stage.

During treatment with 5% guanethidine and 1% adrenaline, added to the maximal therapy of 86 patients with severe glaucoma for a period of 3 years, Romano (1974, 1977) observed an additional drop in IOP of 7 mm Hg or 23%. A 20-50% decrease in IOP could be maintained over a period of 19 months in 60% of the eyes. Treatment was withdrawn because of intolerance in 3 patients. Romano did not observe any more conjunctival hyperaemia with the combination than with adrenaline alone. In one patient there was an annoying ptosis and punctate keratitis was seen occasionally. Surgery could be avoided in 13% of the patients.

The results of the studies described above are rather inconsistent as far as the successfulness and side effects are concerned. They were carried out with 5-10% guanethidine and 0.5-2% adrenaline, the two substances being given separately (guanethidine first).

In addition to the marked decreases in IOP described by various authors, there were many undesirable side effects such as ptosis, conjunctival hyperaemia, swollen eyelids, headache, rhinorrhoea and punctate keratitis. These often led to cessation of treatment. Now, in order to reduce the side effects, the two active principles have been combined into one eyedrop and their concentration has been reduced.

The data from the literature which are presented below pertain to studies with either the combined eyedrops containing 3-5% guanethidine and 0.5-1% adrenaline or with weaker solutions of the two substances given separately.

4.1.2 Guanethidine and adrenaline combined in one eyedrop and the separate application of weaker solutions of the two

The effectiveness of 5% guanethidine and 1% adrenaline, both separately and combined in one eyedrop, was investigated by Jones et al. (1977) in a dose-response study on 18 glaucoma patients. Between 4 and 7 hours

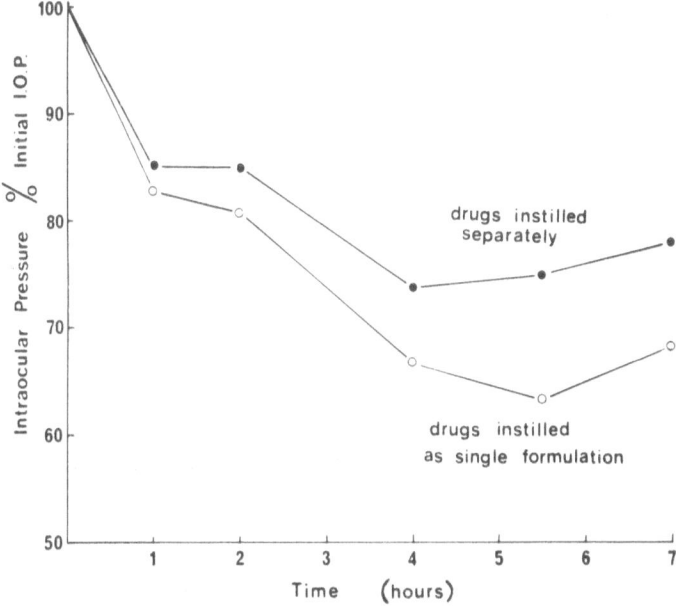

Fig. 12. Effect on intraocular pressure of guanethidine - adrenaline, apart and in one eyedrop, administered on glaucoma patients (by courtesy of Jones et al., 1977).

after application, the combination produced an approximately 10% greater decrease in IOP than the substances applied separately (Fig. 12). In the same way, they compared the combination of 5% guanethidine and 1% adrenaline with a combination of 3% guanethidine and 0.5% adrenaline. The effect on IOP was the same with both combinations, but the side effects were less with the weaker solution.

A double-blind cross-over study with 5% guanethidine, 1% adrenaline and the two agents combined into one eyedrop was carried out by Eltz et al. (1978). During a period of 6 weeks, 63 glaucoma patients were treated with all 3 solutions. The greatest decrease in IOP was observed with the combination of 5% guanethidine and 1% adrenaline, but this also produced the most side effects. Treatment had to be stopped in 8 patients because of intolerance to the combined eyedrop.

A very low dosage was used by Nagasubramian et al. (1976) as supplemental therapy in the treatment of 100 glaucoma patients (181 eyes). In order to reduce the side effects as much as possible, they used a combination of 1% guanethidine and 0.005-0.5% adrenaline in separate eyedrops. Over a period of 6-8 months they observed a satisfactory additional drop in IOP of about 9 mm Hg in 95% of the patients, with no side effects. They concluded that low-dosage therapy with 1% guanethidine and 0.005-0.5% adrenaline is quite useful in the treatment of glaucoma.

In summary, it can be concluded that:
1) guanethidine is able to decrease the IOP by itself, but this effect persists for only a few weeks;
2) the combination of guanethidine and adrenaline produces a greater drop in IOP than either of the two substances separately;
3) there is a definite relationship between dose and response, but that with increasing concentration the number and intensity of the side effects also increases.

4.2 6-Hydroxydopamine and adrenaline in glaucoma simplex

In a study of the supersensitivity to adrenaline after pretreatment with 6-HD, Kitazawa et al. (1972, 1973, 1975) observed an increase in the sensitivity to adrenaline of both pupil and the IOP in normal human and rabbit eyes. The supersensitivity persisted for an average of one month. Glaucoma patients were than given 6-HD by means of iontophoresis and treated with 1% adrenaline eyedrops 3 times a day. In 80% of the cases the IOP dropped to values below 20 mm Hg. They concluded that patients with a moderately elevated IOP respond well to this treatment, but that patients with advanced glaucoma who are already receiving maximal therapy benefit little.

Holland et al. (1973a) treated 92 glaucoma patients for a period of 2 years with subconjunctivally administered 6-HD (0.2 cc) and 1-2% adrenaline 1-3 times a day; the previous treatment was continued if necessary. The best results were obtained in patients with primary open angle glaucoma. In 70% of the glaucoma patients who had not been brought under control by maximal therapy, the IOP decreased to values below 20 mm Hg after treatment with 6-HD and adrenaline. The average decrease in ocular pressure in 128 treated eyes was 13.7 mm Hg or 36.6%.

In addition to treating patients with 6-HD and adrenaline, Holland (1973b, c) investigated the supersensitivity of the glaucomatous eye to adrenaline, phenylephrine and isoproterenol; these studies showed a greatly increased response of the pupil to adrenaline. The sensitivity to adrenaline of the mechanisms responsible for the decrease in IOP, specifically the inhibition of aqueous humor production, was also markedly increased in the denervated eyes. There was no clear potentation of the effect of adrenaline on the mechanisms which regulate the outflow facility. By administering eyedrops containing various concentrations of phenylephrine and isoproterenol to patients who had been treated with 6-HD, they also studied the response of the glaucomatous eye after specific α- and β-adrenergic stimulation. Both the pupil and the IOP were found to be supersensitive to phenylephrine, while with isoproterenol only the IOP could be shown to be supersensitive. The outflow facility was not supersensitive to either phenylephrine or isoproterenol, so that the increased drop in IOP must have been caused by an increased inhibition of aqueous humor production.

In summary, ît appears that pretreatment with 6-HD results in the development of supersensitivity to adrenaline in the mechanisms which regulate the aqueous humor production but not in the mechanisms which regulate the outflow facility. This results in a decrease in IOP.

REFERENCES TO PART ONE

Abadie, C. H. Nature du glaucoma. Explication de l'action curative de l'iridectomie. *Arch. Opthal. (Paris)* 17: *375* (1897).

Ahlquist, R.P. A study of the adrenotropic receptors. *Amer. J. Physiol.* 153: *586* (1948).

Alm, A., Bill, A. & Young, F. A. The effects of pilocarpine and neostigmine in the blood flow through the anterior uvea in monkeys. A study with radio-actively labelled microspheres. *Exp. Eye Res.* 15: *31* (1973).

Alphen van G.W.H.M., Kern, R. & Robinette, S.L. Adrenergic receptors of the intraocular muscles. *Arch. Ophthal.* 74: *253* (1965).

Alphen van, G.W.H.M. & Macri, F.J. Entrance of fluorescein into aqueous humor of cat eye. *Arch. Ophthal.* 75: *247* (1966).

Alphen van, G.W.H.M. The adrenergic receptors of the intraocular muscles of the human eye. *Invest. Ophthal.* 15: *502* (1976).

Anderson, H.K. The paralysis of involuntary muscle, with special reference to the occurence of paradoxical contraction. Part I. Paradoxical pupil-dilation and other phenomena caused by lesions of the cervical sympathetic tract. *J. Physiol.* 30: *290* (1904).

Anderson, H.K. The paralysis of incoluntary muscle. Part III. On the action of pilocarpine, physostigmine, and atropine upon the paralysed iris. *J. Physiol.* 33: *414* (1905-1906).

Anselmi, P., Bron, J. & Maurice, D.M. Action of drugs on the aqueous flow in man measured by fluorophotometry. *Exp. Eye Res.* 7: *487* (1968).

Ariens, E.J. The mode of action in biologically active compounds. In: Molecular Pharmacology. Vol. 1. Academic Press, New York.

Ballantine, E.J. & Garner, L.L. Improvement of the coëfficient of outflow in glaucomatous eyes. *Arch. Ophthal.* 66: *314* (1961).

Balzer, H. & Holtz, P. Beeinflussing der Wirkung biogener Amine durch Hemmung der Aminoxydase. *Arch. Exper. Path. u. Pharmakol.* 227: *547* (1956).

Bárány, E.A. Transient increase in outflow facility after superior cervical ganglionectomy in rabbits. *Arch. Ophthal.* 67: *303* (1962).

Bárány, E.H. & Gnädinger, M.C. Die Wirkung der β-adrenergischen Substanz Isoprenalin auf die Ausfluss-Fazilität des Kaninchenauges. *v. Graefes Arch. Ophthal.* 167: *483* (1964).

Barger, G. & Dale, H.H. Chemical structure and sympathomimetic action of amines. *J. Physiol.* 41: *19* (1910).

Becker, B. & Ley, A.P. Epinephrine and acetazolamide in the therapy of the chronic glaucomas. *Amer. J. Ophthal.* 45: *639* (1958).

Becker, B., Petitt, T.T. & Gay, A.J. Topical epinephrine therapy of open-angle glaucoma. *Arch. Ophthal.* 66: *219* (1961).

Becker, B. & Morton, W. Topical epinephrine in glaucoma suspects. *Amer. J. Ophthal.* 62: *272* (1966).

Bernard, C. Leçons de pathologie experimentale. Paris. J.B. Baillière et fils. 1880.

Bill, A. & Phillips, C.I. Uveoscleral drainage of aqueous humor in human eyes. *Exp. Eye Res.* 12: *275* (1971).

Bill, A. Basic physiology of the drainage of aqueous humor. *Exp. Eye Res. suppl*: 291 (1977).

Bito, L.Z. The physiology of intraocular fluids. *Exp. Eye Res. suppl*: 273 (1977).

Blaschko, H. The specific action of L-dopa decarboxylase. *J. Physiol.* 96: *50* (1939).

Bonomi, L. Sull'azione dell'aleudrina sull'ochio umano normale. *Boll. Oculist.* 43: *112* (1964).

Bonomi, L. & Comite, P. di. Outflow facility after guanethidine sulfate administration. *Arch. Ophthal.* 78: *337* (1967).

Boura, A.L.A. & Green. A.F. Comparison of bretylium and guanethidine: tolerance and effects on adrenergic nerve function and responses to sympathomimetic amines. *Brit. J. Pharmacol.* 19: *13* (1962).

Bron, A.J. Sympathetic control of aqueous secretion in man. *Brit. J. Ophthal.* 53: *37* (1969).

Budge, J.L.Uber die Bewegung der Iris. Vieweg, Branschweig. 125 (1855).

Burn, J.H. The action of tyramine and ephedrine. *J. Pharmacol. Exp. Ther.* 46: *75* (1932).

Burn, J.H. The enzymes at sympathetic nerve endings. *Brit. Med. J.* 1: *784* (1952).

Burn, J.H. & Tainter, M.L. An analysis of the effect of cocaine on the actions of adrenaline and tyramine. *J. Physiol.* 71: *169* (1931).

Burn, J.H. & Rand, M.J. The cause of supersensitivity of smooth muscle to noradrenaline after sympathetic degeneration. *J. Physiol.* 147: *135* (1959).

Cannon, W.B. A law of denervation. *Amer. J. Med. Sc.* 198: *737* (1939).

Castrén, J.A. & Pohjola, S. Effect of guanethidine on glaucomatous eyes. *Acta Ophthal.* 40: *308* (1962).

Castrén, J.A., Pohjola, S., Pakarinen, P. & Karjalainen, K. Guanethidine (Ismeline) in the therapy of glaucoma. *Ophthalmologica* 155: *194* (1968).

Cobb, S. & Scarlett, H. Report of cases of cervical sympathetic nerve injury causing oculopupillary syndrome. *Arch. Neurol. Psychiat.* 3: *636* (1920).

Colasanti, B.K., Chiu, P. & Trotter, R.R. Adrenergic and cholinergic drug effects on rabbit eyes after sympathetic denervation. *Europian J. of Pharm.* 47: *311* (1978).

Colasanti, B.K. & Trotter, R.R. Reduction by hemicholinium-3 of intraocular pressure in the rabbit. *Invest. Ophthalmol. Vis. Sci. ARVO Suppl.* 277 (1979).

Cole, D.F. The site of breakdown of the blood-aqueous barrier under the influence of vaso-dilator drugs. *Exp. Eye Res.* 19: *591* (1974).

Crombie, A.L. Adrenergic hypersensitization as a therapeutic tool in glaucoma. *Trans. Ophthal. Soc. U.K.* 94: *570* (1974).

Crout, J.R. Effect of inhibiting both catechol-O-methyl transferase and monoamine-oxidase on cardiovascular responses to norepinephrine. *Proc. Soc. exp. Bio. N.Y.* 108: *482* (1961).

Csillick, B. Histochemical model experiments on the effects of various drugs on the catecholamine content of adrenergic nerve terminals. *J. Neurochem.* 11: *351* (1964).

Dake, C.L. Glaucoma simplex. A long-term clinical trial. Thesis. Royal van Gorcum and Comp. N.V. 1967.

Dale, H.H. Pharmacology and nerve-endings. *Proc. R. Soc. Med.* 28: *319* (1935).

Dale, H.H. & Feldberg, W. Chemical transmission of secretory impulses to sweat glands of cat. *J. Physiol.* 82: *121* (1934).

Davson, H. The Eye: Vegatative Physiology and Biochemistry. New York. Academic Press Inc. vol. I. 1969.

Docherty, J.R., Mac Donald, A. & Mac Grath, J.C. Further subclassification of α-adrenoceptors in the cardiovascular system, vas deferens and anococcygius of the rat. *Brit. J. Pharmacol.* 67: *421* (1979).

Drance, S.M. The significance of the diurnal tension variations in normal and glaucomatous eyes. *Arch. Ophthal.* 64: *494* (1960).

Drance, S.M. In: Drug Mechanisms in glaucoma. J.A. Churchill, London. pag. 62, 1966.

Drew, G.M. & Whiting, S.B. Evidence for two distinct types of postsynaptic α-adreno-ceptors in vascular smooth muscle in vivo. *Brit. J. Pharmacol.* 67: *207* (1979).

Duke-Elder, S. The anatomy of the visual system. In: System of ophthalmology, Vol. II. *Kimpton London.* 2: *847* (1968).

Eakins, K.E. The effect of intravitreous injections of norepinephrine, epinephrine and isoproterenol on the intraocular pressure and aqueous humor dynamics of rabbits eyes. *J. Pharmacol. Exp. Ther.* 140: *79* (1963).

Eakins, K.E. & Eakins, H.M.T. Adrenergic mechanisms and the outflow of aqueous humor from the rabbit eye. *J. Pharmacol. Exp. Ther.* 144: *60* (1964).

Eakins, K.E. & Ryan, S.J. The action of sympathomimetic amines on the outflow of aqueous humor from the eye. *Brit. J. Pharmacol.* 23: *374* (1964).

Elliot, T.R. The control of the suprarenal glands by the splanchnic nerves. *J. Physiol.* 44: *374* (1912).

Elschnig, A. Irido-ektomie. *Klin. Mbl. Augenheilk.* 50: *538* (1912).

Eltz, H., Aeschliman, J. & Gloor, B. A double-blind clinical trial of a guanethidine-adrenaline combination compared with the two separate components, in glaucoma. *Acta Ophthalmol.* 56: *191* (1978).

Emmelin, N. Supersensitivity following pharmalogical denervation. *Pharmacol. Rev.* 13: *17* (1961).

Etienne, R. The non-miotical topical therapy of glaucoma simplex. A.M.A. Ann. Meeting section Ophthal. 1973.

Euler von, U.S. A specific sympathomimetic ergone in adrenergic nerve fibres (sympathin) and its relations to adrenaline and nor-adrenaline. *Acta Physiol. Scand.* 12: *73* (1946).

Flach, A. J. & Wood, I. An electron micrscopic study of degeneration of nerve terminals after administration of epinephrine. *Exp. Eye Res.* 27: *377* (1978).

Flach, A.J. & Peterson, J.S. Epinephrine nerve terminal degeneration. Invest. Ophthalmol. Vis. Sci. ARVO suppl. 40, 1979.

Fleming, W. W. & Trendelenburg, U. Development of supersensitivity to norepinephrine after pretreatment with reserpine. *J. Pharmacol. Exp. Ther.* 133: *41* (1961).

Fleming, W. W. A comparative study of supersensitivity to norepinephrine and acetylcholine produced by denervation, decentralisation and reserpine. *J. Pharmacol. Exp. Ther.* 141: *173* (1973).

Furchgott, R. F. Receptors for sympathomimetic amines. In: Adrenergic Mechanisms. Churchill Ltd. London. p. 246, 1960.

Gaasterland, D., Kupfer, C., Ross, K. & Gabelnick, H. L. Studies of aqueous humor dynamics in man. III. Measurements in young normal subjects using norepinephrine and isoproterenol. *Invest. Ophthalmol.* 12: *267* (1973).

Garner, L. L., Johnstone, W. W., Ballantine, E. J. & Carroll, M. E. Effect of 2% Levorotary epinephrine on the intraocular pressure of the glaucomatous eye. *Arch. Ophthalmol.* 62: *230* (1959).

Glaubiger, G., Tsai, B. S. & Lefkowitz, R. Chronic guanethidine treatment increases cardiac β-adrenergic receptors. *Nature* 273: *240* (1978).

Gloster, J. Guanethidine and glaucoma. *Trans. Ophthal. Soc. U.K.* 94: *573* (1974).

Gnädinger, M. C. & Bárány, E. H. Die Wirkung der β-adrenergischen Substanz Isoprenalin auf die Ausflusz-Fazilität des Kaninchenauges. *Alb. v. Graefes Arch. Ophthalmol.* 167: *483* (1964).

Goldmann, H. Aubfluszdruck, Minutevolumen und Wirkung der Kammer stromung des Menschen. *Doc. Ophthalmol.* 5-6: *278* (1951).

Gurins, S. & Deluva, A. The biological synthesis of radioactive adrenalin from phenylalanine. *J. Biol. Chem.* 170: *545* (1947).

Hampel, C. W. The effects of denervation on the sensitivity to adrenine of the smooth muscle in the nicitating membrane of the cat. *Amer. J. Physiol.* 111: *611* (1935).

Harris, L. S., Galin, M. A. & Lerner, R. The influence of Low-Dose L-Epinephrine on aqueous outflow facility. *Ann. Ophthal.* 2-5: *455* (1970).

Havener, W. Autonomic drugs. In: Ocular Pharmacology. : 214, 1974. The C.V. Mosby Company.

Hendley, E. & Eakins, K. E. The mechanism of action of guanethidine on aqueous humor dynamics. *J. Pharmacol. Exp. Ther.* 150: *393* (1965).

Hitchings, R. A. & Spaeth, G. L. The optic disc in glaucoma. *Brit. J. Ophthal.* 60: *778* (1976).

Holland, M. G. & Mims, J. L. Anterior segment chemical sympathectomy by 6-hydroxy-dopamine. I. Effect on intraocular pressure and facility of outflow. *Invest. Ophthal.* 10: *120* (1971).

Holland, M. G., Wei, Ch. P. & Gupta, S. Review and evaluation of 6-hydroxydopamine (6-HD): chemical sympathectomy for the treatment of glaucoma. *Ann. Ophthal.* 5-5: *539* (1973a).

Holland, M. G. & Wei, Ch. P. Epinephrine dose-response characteristics of glaucoma-tous human eyes following chemical sympathectomy with 6-hydroxydopamine. *Ann. Ophthal.* 5-6: *633* (1973b).

Holland, M. G. & Wei, Ch. P. Chemical sympathectomy in glaucoma. Therapy: An investigation of alpha and beta adrenergic supersensitivity. *Ann. Ophthal.* 5-7: *783* (1973c).

Holtz, P. Dopadecarboxylase. *Natur Wissenschaften.* 27: *274* (1939).

Horner, J. F. Über ein Form von Ptosis. *Klin. Mbl. Augenheilk.* 7: *193* (1869).

Hoyng, Ph. F. J. & Alphen van, G. W. H. M. Behaviour of IOP and pupil size after topical tranylcypromine in the rabbit eye. *Invest. Ophthalmol. Vis. Sci. ARVO Suppl.* p. 18 (April 1980).

Innemee, H. C. De farmacologische beïnvloeding van de intraoculaire druk via het centrale zenuwstel. Thesis. p. 89 (1979).

Jones, D. E. P., Norton, D. A. & Davies, D. J. G. Low dosage combined adrenaline-guanethidine formulations in the management of chronic simple glaucoma. *Trans. Ophthal. Soc. U. K.* 97: *192* (1977).

Jonnesco, Th. Die Resection des Halssympathicus in der Behandlung des Glaucoma. *Wiener Klinischen Wochenschrift.* 12: *483* (1899).

Kaufman, P. L. Aqueous humor dynamics after total iridectomy in cynomolgus monkeys. *Invest. Ophthalmol. Visc. Sci. ARVO Suppl.* p. 12 (1979).

Kaufman, P. L. & Bárány, E. H. Residual pilocarpine effects on outflow facility after ciliary muscle disinsertion in the cynomolgus monkey. *Invest. Ophthalmol.* 15: *558* (1976a).

Kaufman, P. L. & Bárány, E. H. Loss of acute pilocarpine effect on outflow facility following surgical disinsertion and retrodisplacement of the ciliary muscle from the scleral spur in the cynomolgus monkey. *Invest. Ophthalmol.* 15: *793* (1976b).

Keates, E. U., Krishna, N. & Leopold, I. H. Ocular effects of guanethidine and its use in glaucoma. In symposium on guanethidine. *Memphis: Ciba Pharmaceutical Products Inc.* p. 66 (1960).

Kirpekar, S. M., Cervoni, P. & Furchgott, R. F. Catecholamine content of the cat nictating membrane following procedures sensitizing it to norepinephrine. *J. Pharmacol. Exp. Ther.* 135: *180* (1962).

Kitazawa, Y. Topical adrenergic potentiators in primary open-angle glaucoma. *Amer. J. Ophthal.* 74: *588* (1972).

Kitazawa, Y., Nose, H. & Horie, T. The effect of chemical sympathectomy on intra-ocular pressure of the normal human subjects. *Acta Soc. Ophthal. Jap.* 77: *1901* (1973).

Kitazawa. Y., Nose, H. & Horie, T. Chemical sympathectomy with 6-hydroxydopa-mine in the treatment of primary open-angle glaucoma. *Amer. J. Ophthal.* 79: *98* (1975 a).

Kitazawa, Y. & Horie, T. Diurnal variation of intraocular pressure in primary open angle glaucoma. *Amer. J. Ophthal.* 79: *557* (1975b).

Kopin, L. Biosynthesis and metabolism of catecholamines. *Anesthesiology.* 29: *654* (1968).

Kramer, S. G. & Potts, A. M. Iris uptake of catecholamines in experimental Horner's syndrome. *Amer. J. Ophthal.* 67: *705* (1969a).

Kramer, S. G. & Potts, A. M. Intraocular pressure and ciliary body norepinephrine uptake in experimental Horner's syndrome. *Amer. J. Ophthal.* 68: *1076* (1969b).

Kronfeld, P. C. Dose-effect relationships as an aid in the evaluation of ocular hypotensive drugs. *Invest. Ophthalmol.* 3: *258* (1964).

Küchle, H.J. Zur lokalen Wirkung von Guanethidine (ismeline) auf das gesunde und glaukomkranke Auge. *Klin. Mbl. Augenheilk.* 139: *224* (1961).

Kutschera, E. Klinische Erfahrungen mit Ismelin. *Klin. Mbl. Augenheilk.* 139: *234* (1961).

Lamble, J. W. The effect of topically applied guanethidine sulphate on the pupil and tension responses of the rabbit eye to (−) − adrenaline bitartrate. *Exp. Eye Res.* 19: *79* (1974).

Lands, A. M., Arnold, A., McAuliff, J. P., Luduena, F. P. & Brown, T. G. Differentiation of receptor systems activated by sympathomimetic amines. *Nature* 214: *597* (1967).

Langendorff, O. Der Deuting der 'paradoxen' Pupillenerweiterung. *Klin. Mbl. Augenheilk.* 38: *823* (1900).

Langer, S. Z. Presynaptic regulation of catecholamine release. *Biochem. Pharmac.* 23: *1793* (1974).

Langham, M. E. & Taylor, C. B. The effect of superior cervical ganglionectomy on the intraocular pressure. *J. Physiol.* 147: *58* (1959).

Langham, M. E. & Taylor, C. B. The influence of pre- and postganglionic section of the cervical sympathetic on the intraocular pressure of rabbits and cats. *J. Physiol.* 152: *437* (1960a).

Langham, M. E. & Taylor, C. B. The influence of superior cervical ganglionectomy on intraocular dynamics. *J. Physiol.* 152: *447* (1960b).

Langham, M. E. & Rosenthal, R. The influences of electrical stimulation of the preganglionic superior cervical sympathetic nerve on the secretion of aqueous humor and the intraocular pressure in rabbits. *Fed. Proc.* 23: *517* (1964).

Langham, M. E. & Rosenthal, R. The role of the cervical sympathetic nerve in the regulation of the intraocular pressure and circulation. *Amer. J. Physiol.* 210: *786* (1966).

Langham. M. E. & Weinstein, G. W. Horner's syndrome. Ocular supersensitivity to adrenergic amines. *Arch. Ophthalmol.* 78: *462* (1967).

Langham, M. E., Kitazawa, Y. & Hart, R. W. Adrenergic responses in the human eye. *J. Pharm. Exp. Ther.* 179: *47* (1971).

Langham, M. E. & Diggs, E. β-Adrenergic Responses in the eyes of rabbits, primates and man. *Exp. Eye Res.* 19: *281* (1974).

Leydhecker, W. Glaukom. Ein Handbuch. p. 410, 1973. Springer Verlag. Zweite auflage.

Linksz, A. Der Einfluss der Sympathicus Ausschaltung auf die Blut-Kammerwasserschranke. *Klin. Wschr.* 10: *839* (1931).

Loewi, O. & Navratil, E. Über humorale Übertragbarkeit der Herznervenwirkung. Mitteilung über das Schicksal des Vagusstoff. *Pflügers Arch. ges. Physiol.* 214: *678* (1926).

Luco, J. V. The sensitizations of inhibited structures by denervation. *Amer. J. Physiol.* 120: *179* (1937).

Macri, F. J. & Cevario, S. J. Ciliary ganglion stimulation: I. Effects on aqueous humor inflow and outflow. *Invest. Ophthalmol.* 14: *28* (1975).

Macri, F. J. & Cevario, S. J. The formation and inhibition of aqueous humor production. A proposed mechanism of action. *Arch. Ophthalmol.* 96: *1664* (1978).

Mantegazza, P., Tyler, C. & Zaimis, E. The peripheral action of hexamethonium and of pentolinium. *Brit. J. Pharmacol.* 13: *480* (1958).

Maxwell, R. A., Plummer, A. J., Schneider, F., Povalki, H. & Daniel, A. I. Pharmacology of [2- (octahydro-1-azocinyl)- Ethyl] – guanidine sulfate (SU-5864). *J. Pharmacol. Exp. Ther.* 128: *22* (1960a).

Maxwell, R. A., Plummer, A. J., Povalski, H. & Schneider, F. Concerning a possible action of guanethidine (SU-5864) in smooth muscle. *J. Pharmacol. Exp. Ther.* 129: *24* (1960b).

Meltzer, S. J. & Meltzer Auer, C. Studies on the 'Paradoxical' pupil-dilatation caused by adrenalin. I. The effect of subcutaneous injections and instillations of adrenalin upon the pupils of rabbits. *Amer. J. Physiol.* 11: *28* (1904).

Meltzer, S. J. Studies on the 'Paradoxical' pupil-dilitation caused by adrenalin. II. On the influence of subcutaneous injections of adrenalin upon the eyes of cats after removal of the superior cervical ganglion. *Amer. J. Physiol.* 11: *37* (1904).

Merté, H. J. & Toppel, L. Guanethidine in der Glaukomtherapie. *Albrecht v. Graefes Arch. Klin. Exp. Ophthal.* 176: *30* (1968).

Miller, S.J.H. Stellate ganglion blockade in glaucoma. *Brit. J. Ophthal.* 37: *70* (1953).

Mitchell, J. R. & Oates, J. A. Guanethidine and related agents. 1. Mechanism of the selective blockade of adrenergic neurons and its antagonism by drugs. *J. Pharm. Exp. Ther.* 172: *100* (1970).

Moses, R. A. The iris and the pupil. Adler's Physiology of the eye, 6th edition. *Moses Ed., Saint Louis, USA.* 320 (1975).

Nagasubramanian, S., Tripathi, R. C., Poinoosawmy, D. & Gloster, J. Low concentration guanethidne and adrenaline therapy of glaucoma. A preliminary report. *Trans. Ophthal. Soc. U.K.* 96: *179* (1976).

Neufeld, A. H., Chavis, R. M. & Sears, M. L. Degeneration release of norepinephrine causes transient ocular hyperemia mediated by prostaglandins. *Invest. Ophthal.* 12: *167* (1973).

Neufeld, A., Dueker, D.K., Vegge, T. & Sears, M.L. Adenosine 3'-5' monophosphate increases the outflow of aqueous humor from the rabbit eye. *Invest. Ophthalmol.* 14: *40* (1975a).

Neufeld, A.H. & Sears, M.L. Adenosine 3'-5'-monophosphate analogue increases the outflow facility of the primate eye. *Invest. Ophthalmol.* 14/9: *688* (1975b).

Neufeld, A. Influence of cyclic nucleotides on outflow facility in the vervet monkey. *Exp. Eye Res.* 27: *387* (1978).

Neufeld, A. H., Zawistowski, K. A., Page, E. D. & Bromberg, B. B. Influences on the density of β-adrenergic receptors in the cornea and iris-ciliary body of the rabbit. *Invest. Ophthalmol.* 17: *1072* (1978).

Obstbaum, S. A., Kolker, A. E. & Phelps, Ch. D. Low-Dose Epinephrine. Effect on intraocular pressure. *Arch. Ophthal.* 92: *118* (1974).

Oosterhuis, J. A. Guanethidine (ismeline) in Ophthalmology. 1. Observations in rabbits. *Arch. Ophthal.* 67: *592* (1966a).

Oosterhuis, J.A. Guanethidine (ismeline) in Ophthalmology. 2. Clinical application in glaucoma. *Arch. Ophthal.* 67: *802* (1966b).

Page, E. D. & Neufeld, A. H. Characterization of α- and β-adrenergic receptors in membranes prepared from the rabbit iris before and after development of supersensitivity. *Biochem. Pharmacol.* 27: *953* (1978).

Paterson, G. D. & Paterson, G. Drug therapy of glaucoma. *Brit. J. Ophthal.* 56: *288* (1972).

Paterson, G. D., Paterson, G. & Miller, S. H. J. The non-miotic therapy of open angle glaucoma. *Internat. Glauc. Symp. Albi.* p. 343 (1974).

Podos, S. M., Becker, B. & Kass, M. A. Prostaglandin synthesis, inhibition and intraocular pressure. *Invest. Ophthal.* 12: *426* (1974).

Pollack, I. P. Effect of L-norepinephrine and adrenergic potentiators on the aqueous humor dynamics of man. *Amer. J. Ophthal.* 76: *641* (1973).

Pollack, I. P. & Rossi, H. Norepinephrine in treatment of ocular hypertension and glaucoma. *Arch. Ophthal.* 93: *173* (1975).

Porter, C. C., Totaro, J. A. & Stone, C. A. Effects of some dopamine derivates upon tissue catecholamines. *Pharmacol.* 4: *149* (1962).

Richardson, K. C. The fine structure of the albino rabbit iris with special reference to the identification of adrenergic and cholinergic nerves and nerve-endings in its intrinsic muscles. *Am. J. Anat.* 114: *173* (1964).

Richardson, K. T. Autonomic Pharmacology. *Symp. Ocular Pharm. Ther.* p. 32 (1970).

Richardson, K. T. Sympathetic physiology and pharmacology. *Surv. of Ophthalmol.* 17: *120* (1972).

Romano, J. Trial with guanethidine 5% and neutrial adrenaline 1% in eyes with advanced glaucoma. *Trans. Ophthal. Soc. U.K.* 94: *576* (1974).

Romano, J. Use of guanethidine 5 per cent and adrenaline 1 per cent in the treatment of severe open angle glaucoma. *Trans. Ophthal. Soc. U.K.* 97: *196* (1977).

Rosenblueth, A. The actions of certain drugs on the nictating membrane. *Amer. J. Physiol.* 100: *443* (1932).

Ross, R. A. & Drance, S. M. Effects of topically applied isoproterenol on aqueous dynamics in man. *Arch. Ophthal.* 83: *39* (1970).

Roth, J. A. Guanethidine and adrenaline used in combination in chronic simple glaucoma. *Brit. J. Ophthal.* 57: *507* (1973).

Schwartz, C. Cupping and pallor of the optic disc. *Arch. Ophthalmol.* 89: *272* (1973).

Sears, M. L. & Bárány, E. H. Outflow resistance and adrenergic mechanisms. *Arch. Ophthalmol.* 64: *839* (1960).

Sears, M. L. & Sherk, T. E. Supersensitivity of aqueous outflow resistance in rabbits after sympathetic denervation. *Nature.* 11: *387* (1963).

Sears, M. L. & Sherk, T. E. The trabecular effect of noradrenaline in the rabbit eye. *Invest. Ophthalmol.* 3: *157* (1964).

Sears, M. L. The mechanism of action of adrenergic drugs in glaucoma. *Invest. Ophthalmol.* 5: *115* (1966).

Sears, M. L. & Gillis, C. N. Mydriasis and the increase in outflow of aqueous humor from the rabbit eye after cervical ganglionectomy in relation to the release of norepinephrine from the iris. *Bioch. Pharmacol.* 16: *359* (1967).

Shen, S. C. & Cannon, W. B. Sensitization of the denervated pupillary sphincter to acetylcholine. *Chinese J. Physiol.* 10: *359* (1936).

Sonntag, J. R., Brindly, G. O. & Shields, M. B. Effect of timolol therapy on outflow facility. *Invest Ophthalmol.* 17: *293* (1978).

Sonntag, J. R., Brindley, G. O., Shields, B., Nour-Iddin, T. A. & Phelps, Ch. D. Timolol and Epinephrine. Comparison of efficacy and side effects. *Arch. Ophthalmol.* 97: *273* (1979).

Starke, K. & Langer, S. Z. A note on terminology for presynaptic receptors. In: Presynaptic Receptors Adv, in the Biosciences. *Pergamon Press Oxford.* 18: *1* (1979).

Stepanik, J. Tonografische und differential tonometrische Untersuchungen über die Wirkung von Ismelin-Augentropfen bei Glaucoma Simplex. *Alb. v. Graefes Arch. Ophthalmol.* 164: *6* (1961).

Sutherland, E. W. & Rall, T. W. The relation of adenosine-3-5-phosphate and phosphorylase to the actions of catecholamines and other hormones. *Pharmacol. Rev.* 12: *265* (1960).

Swegmark, G. Aqueous humor dynamics in Horner's syndrome. *Trans. Ophthal. SOc. U.K.* 83: *255* (1963).

Tamura, T. Effects of guanethidine on the vesiculated axon in the dilator muscle area of the rabbit iris: An electron microscopical study. *Japan J. Ophthal.* 17: *140* (1973).

Timmermans, P. B. M. W. M., Kwa, H. Y. & Zwieten van, P. A. Possible subdivision of postsympatic α-adrenoceptors mediating pressor responses in the pithed rat. *Naumyn Schmiedebergs Arch. Pharmacol.* 310: *189* (1979).

Towsend, D. J. & Brubaker, R. F. Immediate effect of epinephrine on aqueous formation in the normal human eye as measured by fluorophotometry. *Invest. Ophthalmol. Vis. Sci.* 19: *256* (1980).

Tranzer, J.P., Thoenen, H. An electron microscopic study of selective, acute degeneration of sympathetic nerve terminals after administration of 6-Hydroxydopamine. *Experientia* 24: *155* (1968).

Tregubova, R. S. The influence of ornide on intraocular pressure in glaucomatous patients. *Zentralblatt.* 99: *79* (1967).

Treister, G. & Bárány, E. The effect of bretylium on the degeneration mydriasis and intraocular pressure decrease in the conscious rabbit after unilateral cervical ganglionectomy. *Invest. Ophthalmol.* 9: *343* (1970).

Trendelenburg, U. & Weiner, N. Sensitivity of the nictating membrane to various sympathomimetic amines. *J. Pharmacol. Exp. Ther.* 138: *181* (1962).

Trendelenburg, U. Supersensitivity and subsensitivity to sympathomimetic amines. *Pharmac. Rev.* 15: *225* (1963).

Trendelenburg, U. Mechanisms of supersensitivity and subsensitivity to sympathomimetic amines. *Pharma. Rev.* 18/1: *629* (1966).

Veldstra, H. Synergism and potentiation with special reference to the combination of structural analogues. *Pharmacol. Rev.* 8: *339* (1956).

Vernikos-Danellis, J. & Zaimis, E. Some pharmacological actions of bretylium and guanethidine. *Lancet,* ii: *787* (1960).

Waltman, S. & Sears, M. L. Catechol-O-methyl transferase in the ocular tissues of albino rabbits. *Invest. Ophthalmol.* 3: *601* (1964).

Wand, M. & Grant, W. M. Thymoxamine hydrochloride: effects on the facility of outflow and intraocular pressure. *Invest. Ophthal.* 15: *400* (1976).

Wand, M. & Grant, W. M. Thymoxamine Test. Differentiating angle-course glaucoma from open-angle glaucoma with narrow angles. *Arch. Ophthalmol.* 96: *1009* (1978).

Weekers, R., Prijot, E. & Gustin, J. Mode d'action de l'adrenaline dans le glaucoma chronique. *Ophthalmologica (Basel).* 128: *213* (1954).

Weisman, R. L., Assef, C. F., Phelps, Ch. D., Podos, S. M. & Becker, B. Vertical elongation of the optic cup in glaucoma. *Trans. Am. Acad. Ophthalmol. Otolaryngol.* 77: *157* (1973).

Wikberg, J. E. S. Pharmacological classification of adrenergic α-receptors in the guinea pig. *Nature* 273: *164* (1978).

Wikberg, J. E. S. Differentiation between pre- and postjunctional α-receptors in guinea pig ileum and rabbit aorta. *Acta Physiol. Scand.* 103: *225* (1978).

Wilke, K. Early effects of epinephrine and pilocarpine on the intraocular pressure and the episcleral venous pressure in the normal human eye. *Acta Ophthal.* 52: *231* (1974).

Wolf, M. Wirkung von guanethidine 10% auf die Blutkammerwasserschranke. *D.O.G.* 70: *551* (1969).

Zimmerman, T. J. Timolol and facility of outflow. *Invest. Ophthalmol.* 16: *623* (1977).

PART TWO

CLINICAL INVESTIGATIONS

CHAPTER V

INTRODUCTION TO PART II

5.1 Patients and methods

The investigation was carried out on an ambulatory basis in all patients. All patients had been referred to the glaucoma department of the Univeristy Eye Clinic in Amsterdam by other ophthalmologists for evaluation and treatment of elevated intraocular pressure (IOP). In all patients who took part in one of the studies, both an ophthalmological and a general case history were taken. Any ophthalmological treatments which had been given in the past were recorded, together with the general therapy. Patients who were under treatment with beta-blockers, α-methyldopa, reserpine, ismelin or tricyclic antidepressants were excluded from the study. All patients either had primary open angle glaucoma (POAG) or were glaucoma suspects.

A patient was regarded as having POAG if the average IOP in a daycurve without medication was over 22 mm Hg, with either a visual field defect or a pathologically excavated optic disc or both, and with an open angle.

A patient was suspected of having glaucoma if the average IOP in a daycurve without treatment was over 22 mm Hg, with a normal visual field and optic disc, with no IOP over 36 mm Hg and with an open angle. If one eye had glaucoma and the fellow eye showed only an elevated IOP, then both eyes were regarded as having POAG.

The ophthalmological examination included measurement of visual acuity and refraction, evaluation of the anterior segment with the Haag-Streit slitlamp and ophthalmoscopy. Gonioscopy was performed under normal conditions and in mydriasis using Goldmann's three-mirror contact-glass and the condition of the papilla and blood vessels was evaluated binocularly in mydriasis. The visual field examination consisted of both kinetic and static perimetry.

In all patients, treatment was stopped at least 48 hours earlier if they were on miotics and a week before the beginning of the study if they were receiving sympathomimetics or carbonic anhydrase inhibitors. A daycurve without medication was then recorded, the measurements (at least 4) being taken at 9.00 and 12.00 a.m. and 3.00 and 5.00 p.m. Subsequently, treatment was started and daycurves during treatment were recorded. In addition, all patients were followed up at intervals of one or two months, at which time the visual acuity, refraction, anterior segment and IOP were evaluated and the patients were questioned about (and examined for) side effects.

At the end of the study the visual field examination was repeated, the IOP was determined using a Goldmann tonometer mounted on a Haag-Streit slit-lamp, the diameter of the pupil was measured under standardized conditions (31.5 Asb) using the measuring ocular in the Goldmann perimeter, and tonography was performed using the electronic tonograph of Mueller.

Other treatment was avoided during the study as much as possible in order to isolate the effects on the eye and the IOP of the compounds under investigation. The study was carried out with a combination of 3% guanethidine and 0.5% adrenaline in one eyedrop (SUPREXON 3-0.5, Dispersa) and with a combination of 1% guanethidine and 0.2% adrenaline in one eyedrop (SUPREXON 1-0.2, Dispersa). Unless otherwise indicated the combination was applied twice daily (at 9.00 a.m. and 9.00 p.m.).

5.2 Personal investigation

As indicated previously, the study extended over a period of 4 years (1976-1979). It involved a total of 68 patients, some of whom were in several investigations while others participated only a single long-term study.

The first investigation was a double-blind study of the effect of a single drop of 3% guanethidine + 0.5% adrenaline in a group of 19 patients (Ch. VI).

This was followed by a long-term study (7 months) with 3% guanethidine − 0.5% adrenaline twice daily in 33 patients (Ch. VII). During this study the relationship between dilation of the pupil and the course of the IOP after 3% guanethidine − 0.5% adrenaline was also investigated (Ch. IX). One of the reasons this was done is because a biphasic response of the IOP had been noted during the treatment (Ch. VIII). The nature of this biphasic response was also analyzed further (Ch. X).

Since the literature (see Ch. III) concerning the effect of guanethidine alone on the aqueous humor dynamics in glaucoma patients is unclear and the effect of the combination of guanethidine and adrenaline on the aqueous humor dynamics had not yet been investigated, during the long-term study a group of POAG patients and a group of glaucoma suspects were also followed tonographically and the results in the two groups were compared (Ch XI).

Finally, at the end of the long-term study with 3% guanethidine − 0.5% adrenaline, the possibility of applying this combination only once a day was investigated over a period of 4 months in 24 glaucoma patients (Ch. XII). The results obtained were compared with those of twice daily application.

The report of personal research ends with the long-term results obtained with the twice daily application of 1% guanethidine – 0.2% adrenaline in 31 patients (Ch. XIII). Here again, supplemental treatment was avoided. In every chapter of part II, the methods used are described in detail.

5.3 Comments

5.3.1 Comment on the daycurves

The IOP is not constant but shows diurnal fluctuations, also in normal subjects. In view of the spontaneous variations in IOP, the recording of an IOP curve with and without medication is necessary in order to be able to evaluate the effects of the treatment being tested. Ideally, these should be diurnal curves (extending over 24 hours), but this is impossible in a large group of patients for practical reasons. Although some authors (Drance, 1960; Leydhecker, 1973) have reported that 60% of the highest IOP's in glaucoma are seen outside of office hours, Kitazawa (1975) maintains that most of the IOP maxima do fall within the working day. We have limited ourselves to daycurves extending from 9.00 a.m. to 5.00 p.m. and based on at least 4 measurements of the IOP (at 9.00 a.m. and 12.00 a.m. and 3.00 and 5.00 p.m.). It was, however, possible to measure the IOP 12-20 hours (or 16-24 hours) after the last medication since the patient could be asked to apply the last drops at 9.00 p.m. (or 5.00 p.m.) on the day before the study.

5.3.2 Comment on the examination of the optic disc

One of the criteria for determining whether a patient has suspected glaucoma or established glaucoma is cupping of the optic disc. The process of tissue loss leading from a normal disc to a pathologically excavated one is gradual and it is a well-known fact that different experienced investigators can have divergent opinions about the same glaucomatous disc. The criteria used during examination of the optic disc were in accordance with those reported by Schwartz (1973), Weisman et al. (1973) and Hitchings and Spaeth (1976). The pathological aspects which were looked at closely included: asymmetry of the two optic discs, a cup-disc ratio above 0.6 in the vertical meridian or a difference in cupping of 0.2 or more, pallor and thinning of the neuroretinal rim, displacement of the papillary vessels due to focal tissue loss (notching) or general loss with bayoneting of the vessels, exposure of the cribrosa structure with steepening of the walls of the cup, and evidence of slits and wedges in the nerve fiber layer examined under redfree light.

5.3.3 Comment on the visual field examination

Patients who took part in the study were subjected to kinetic perimetry with Goldmann perimeter and static perimetry with the Friedman V.F.A. and Tübingen perimeter. Static perimetry is of the most value during long-term treatment of glaucoma due to the central 30° field. If perimetry is carried out accurately and regularly, then progression can be detected in an early stage so that surgery or some other form of treatment can be resorted to on time.

5.3.4 Comment concerning tonography

The results of tonography as an investigative technique for the early diagnosis of glaucoma and the evaluation of a therapeutic effect in the individual patient have been disappointing due to the many variables which must be taken into consideration. However, the method has proven quite useful for studies on the long-term effects of drugs in groups of patients.

CHAPTER VI

A Double-Blind Short-Term Trial of Guanethidine 3 % and Adrenaline 0.5 % Combined in One Eye Drop

Ph.F.J. Hoyng, C.L. Dake, and E.L. Greve

Summary. A double-blind short-term trial was done to test the effect of guane-thidine 3% – adrenaline 0.5% (G–A) in a combined eye drop in 18 patients with open-angle glaucoma and one patient with narrow-angle glaucoma. In 9 of the 19 patients we expected an IOP lowering agent. There was one false-negative result. The mean fall in IOP due to G–A was 10.1 mm Hg (range 3 to 23) and 8.7 mm Hg (range −1 to 26) 6 and 8 h after application respectively. There was no effect on IOP in the 9 eyes that received the placebo.

Introduction

For more than a century supersensitivity after denervation or decentralization has been a well-known phenomenon in the physiology and pharmacology of the eye (Budge, 1855; Hampel, 1935; Cannon, 1939; Emmelin, 1961; Trendelenburg, 1963). Sears (1966) showed in studies on patients with Horners' syndrome "that the outflow me-chanism can be made supersensitive to topical epinephrine."

Adrenergic supersensitivity after pharmacologic denervation with guanethidine in long-term studies on glaucoma simplex patients has been tested with good results in lowering the intraocular pressure (IOP) in man, though there were many side effects (Paterson and Paterson, 1972; Paterson et al., 1974; Roth, 1973; Collignon and Pryot, 1973; Etienne, 1973; Crombi, 1974; Gloster, 1974; Romano, 1974; Nagasubramanian et al., 1976).

The concentrations used were between 0.05 and 2% adrenaline and between 1 and 10% guanethidine. Paterson and Paterson (1972) found a 9.7 ± 1.1 mm Hg IOP lowering effect of 3% guanethidine alone. However, after 1 month IOP returned to normal or even above normal. The combination of 3% guanethidine with 1% adrenaline produced a 30% fall in the IOP which was even greater between 6 and 12 months of therapy. There was no different effect on IOP with 0.5% adrenaline instead of 1% adrenaline (Paterson et al., 1974). Before starting a longterm study with a combined eye drop of guanethidine 3% – adrenaline 0.5% (G–A) we tested its short-term effect in a double-blind study on 18 patients with open-angle glaucoma and one patient with narrow-angle glaucoma.

Material and Methods

Two eye drops were used, one containing 3% guanethidine − 0.5% adrenaline and the other containing only the vehicle. The second drop was used as placebo.

G−A is an approximately isotonic solution of adrenalin 0.5%, guanethidine 3.0% with N-acetyl cysteine added as anti- oxydant. This solution has a pH 6.5 and has also a good stability provided it is packaged under nitrogen and suitably protected from the atmospheric oxygen. (Zyma Z-15000) Both the active solution and the placebo were supplied in identical bottles, each labeled with a number. The examiner did not know the content of each separate bottle. The key to the code was not received until all examinations were finished. There were 19 patients who entered the study (10 males, 9 females), between 48 and 81 years of age.

In this group were 14 patients with established glaucoma and a wide angle, 4 glaucoma suspects with a wide angle and 1 patient with chronic narrow-angle glaucoma.

Patients on pilocarphine or glaucostat® stopped their current medication 2 days before the trial and patients on daranide ®, diamox ®, isopto-epinal ®, eppy ®, or glaucadrine ® stopped their medication 1 week before the trial. Biomicroscopy was done with a Haag-Streit Slitlamp and the chamber angle was evaluated with a three-mirror contact glass from Goldmann.

IOP was measured with a Goldmann applanation tonometer. We made one diurnal IOP curve without therapy and on the following day a diurnal IOP curve with G−A or the placebo in the eye with the highest IOP found in the first diurnal curve. IOP was measured at 9, 10.30, and 12 a.m. and at 3 and 5 p.m. (0−1 1/2−3−6−8 h after application). On the second day one drop of G−A or its placebo was given 5 min after the first IOP reading and the fellow eye was used as a control.

Results

After evaluation of the results we surmised that 9 out of 19 bottles contained an active agent and 10 a placebo.

After receiving the code we found that all these 9 bottles indeed contained G−A. However, 1 of the remaining 10 bottles in which we suspected a placebo actually contained G−A. The reduction of IOP after 1 1/2−3−6−8 h was statistically evaluated. The IOP of the G−A treated eyes was significantly lower than that of the untreated fellow eyes (paired t-test, $P < 0.01$). Table 1 shows the results. The diurnal IOP curves without medication of the 10 eyes that were to receive G−A on the second day are represented in Figure 1. The 10 diurnal IOP curves with G−A are represented in Figure 2. Figures 3 and 4 represent the means of the IOP differences of 10 G−A treated eyes in mm Hg and percent respectively. The mean results of the untreated fellow eyes are also indicated (*dotted line*).

Other effects of G−A were the following:
Two patients had hyperemia of the conjunctiva bulbi 6 h after application; two pa-

Table 1. Data for treated and untreated diurnal IOP curves, and for the diurnal IOP curves of the fellow (control) eyes

Time after the first measurement (h)	0	1 1/2	3	6	8
Mean IOP, 10 eyes without G—A (mm Hg)	27.7	27.8	28.9	27.4	25.8
Mean IOP, 10 eyes with one drop G—A (mm Hg)	25.8	22.0	24.4	17.3	17.1
Mean IOP diff. of 10 G—A treated eyes (mm Hg)	−1.9	−5.8	−4.5	−10.1	−8.7
Median percent IOP diff. of 10 G—A treated eyes	−10%	−23.5%	−21%	−35%	−37%
Mean IOP, 10 fellow eyes without G—A (mm Hg)	25.1	25.1	25.5	23.6	23.2
Mean IOP, 10 fellow eyes on the day of G—A (mm Hg)	23.6	24.4	25.1	23.2	24.2
Mean IOP diff. of 10 fellow eyes (mm Hg)	−1.5	−0.7	−0.4	−0.4	+0.8

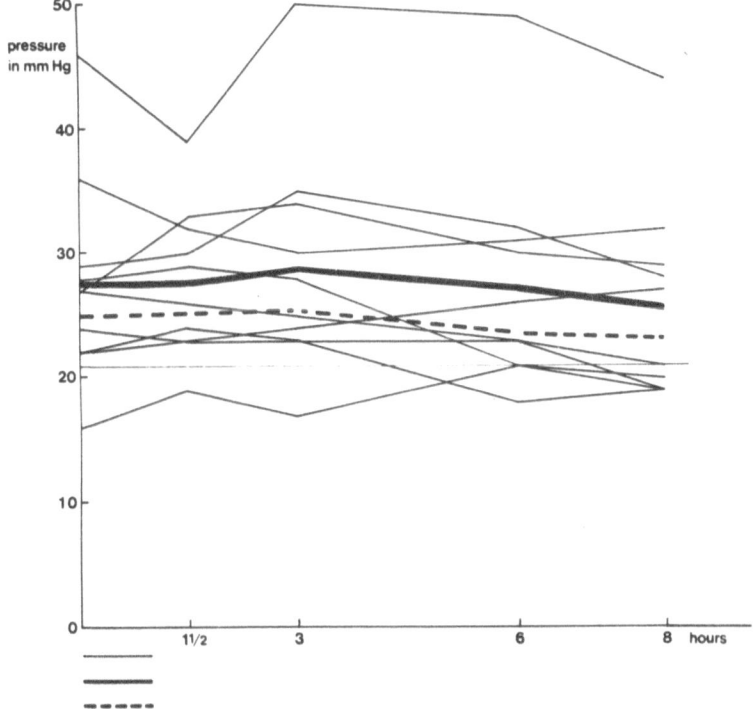

Fig. 1. Diurnal IOP curves of 10 glaucomatous eyes to be treated with G—A without medication (*solid line*) and their mean diurnal IOP curve (*heavy line*). Mean diurnal IOP curve of 10 fellow eyes on the same day (*dotted line*). Abscissa: time after application. Ordinate: IOP in mm Hg

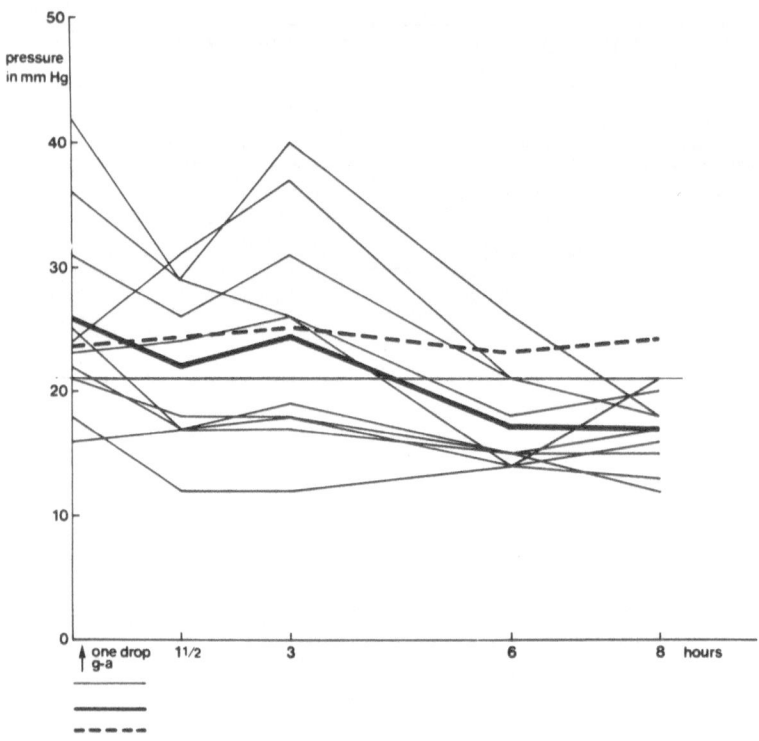

Fig. 2. Diurnal IOP curves of 10 glaucomatous eyes treated with one drop G—A (*solid line*); their mean diurnal curve (*heavy line*) and the mean diurnal IOP curve of 10 fellow eyes on the same day (*dotted line*). Application at time zero. Abscissa: time after application. Ordinate: IOP in mm Hg

tients complained of burning eyes in the 15 to 30 min after application; in one patient there was a narrowing of the interpalpebral fissure 8 h after application and moderate mydriasis occurred in 4 patients.

The IOP of the 9 eyes treated with a placebo was not significantly lowered. No other effects like hyperemia or mydriasis were seen.

Comment

Guanethidine initially removes the noradrenalin from the granulated vesicles in the axoplasma of the sympathic nerve ends. Guanethidine is thought to be taken up by the same membrane transport system as noradrenalin (Mitchel and Oats, 1970). The reuptake of noradrenalin (normally 90%) is blocked and a depletion of noradrenalin

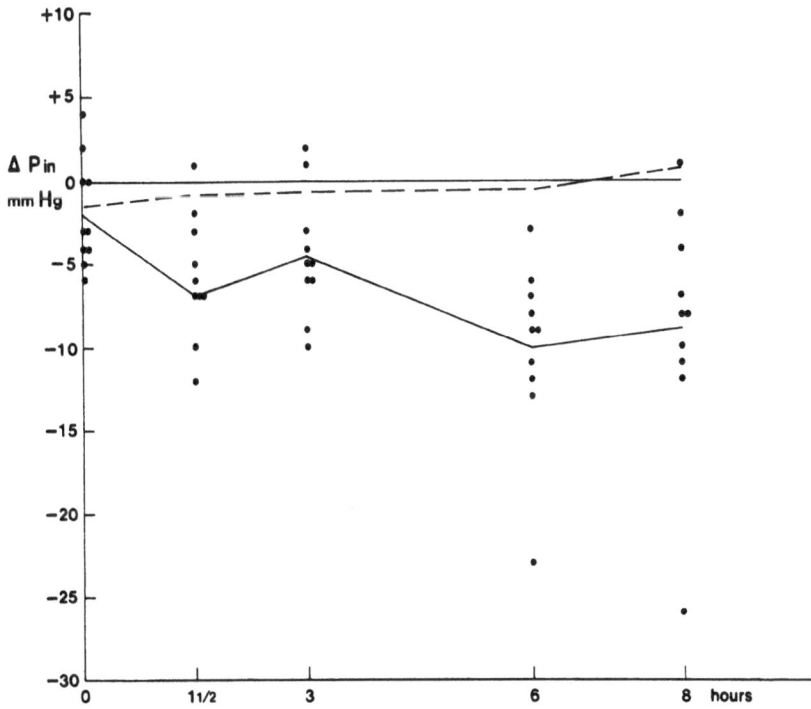

Fig. 3. The mean difference between the diurnal IOP curves without treatment and after treatment with G—A (*solid line*). The *dotted line* indicates the mean IOP curves of the 10 fellow (control) eyes. Application at time zero. Abscissa: time after application. Ordinate: Δ P in mm Hg

in the axoplasma results (Tamura, 1973). At this time supersensitivity at the effector site for adrenergic medication develops. The initial fall in IOP with guanethidine is due to increased outflow (Stepanic, 1961; Kutschera, 1961; Hendley and Eakins, 1965) and after 12 h also to an inhibition of aqueous production (Bonomi and di Comite, 1967). Castren and Pohjala (1962) and Castren et al. (1968) studied dose response curves on patients treated with 5% guanethidine. They found an average decrease in IOP of 9 mm Hg or 37%. The maximum was reached 7 h after application.

Adrenaline has an initial effect on IOP by lowering the aqueous production within 2 h after topical application. This effect is overlapped by increased outflow facility (α-adrenergic effect) which reaches its maximum within 4—6 h. (Weekers et al., 1954; 1955; Becker and Ley, 1958; Gardner et al., 1959).
Weekers et al. (1955) found a fall of 8.5 mm Hg after levo-adrenaline 2%.

Garner et al. (1959) found in 44 glaucomatous eyes an average fall in IOP of 13.5 mm Hg after installation of one drop of 2% solution of levo-adrenaline. The maximum fall in IOP was reached after 4 h.

Other investigators (Harris et al., 1970) found an IOP lowering effect by adrenaline 0.5% of 4.64 ± 0.56 mm Hg after 2 weeks and 5.00 ± 0.52 mm Hg after 4 weeks of treatment (twice a day).

Our study of the effect on IOP of a combination of guanethidine 3% and adrenaline 0.5% was based on a double-blind one-eye treatment using the other eye as a control.

We found an average IOP lowering effect of 10.1 mm Hg (range 3 to 23 mm Hg) or 35% (median percent pressure difference range 6 to 47%) 6 h after application of one drop G—A and 8.7 mm Hg (range −1 to 26 mm Hg) or 37% (median percent pressure difference range −5 to 59%) 8 h after application of one drop G—A.

These data are comparable with the data for guanethidine 5% alone (Castren and Pohjala, 1962; Castren et al., 1968) and for guanethidine 3% alone (Paterson and Paterson, 1972). It seems therefore that the initial effect of G—A is due to guane-thidine 3% alone. Adrenaline 0.5% alone gives an IOP lowering effect of ± 4.5 mm Hg. The IOP lowering effect of G—A in the single-dose diurnal IOP curve is probably the

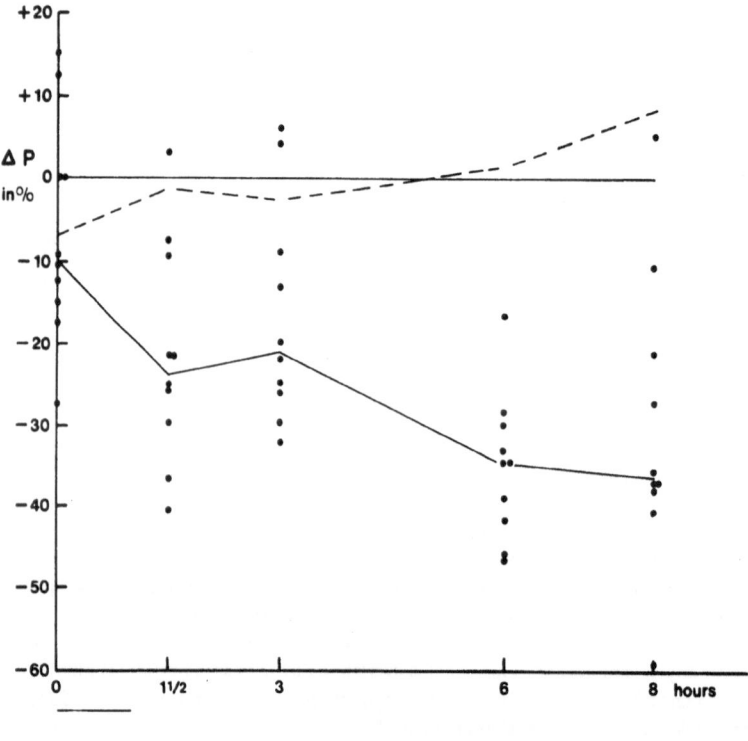

Fig. 4. The median percent difference between the diurnal IOP curves without treatment and after treatment with G—A (*solid line*). The *dotted line* indicates the difference between the 2 diurnal IOP curves of 10 untreated fellow eyes. Application at time zero. Abscissa: time after application. Ordinate: Δ P in %

result of the noradrenaline initially removed from its stores in the axoplasma of the symphathetic nerve ends by guanethidine and not yet the result of supersensitivity.

Therefore a single-dose diurnal IOP curve is not the ideal set-up to evaluate the effect on IOP of drugs that induce supersensitivity.

Acknowledgement. We gratefully acknowledge the skillful assistance ot Mr. W.H. Miller.

References

Becker, B., Ley, A.P.: Epinephrine and acetazolamide. Amer. J. Ophthal. 45, 639–643 (1958)

Bonomi, L., di Comite, P.: Outflow facility after guanethidine sulfate administration. Arch. Ophthal. 78, 337–340 (1967)

Budge, J.: Über die Bewegung der Iris. Braunschweig: Vieweg 1855

Cannon, W.B.: A law of denervation. Amer. J. med. sci. 198, 737–750 (1939)

Castrén, J.A., Pohjala, S.: Effect of guanethidine on glaucomatous eyes. Acta Ophthal. (Kbh) 40, 308–312 (1962)

Castrén, J.A., Pohjala, S., Pakarinen, P., Karjalainen, K.: Guanethidine (Ismelin) in the therapy of glaucoma. Ophthalmologica (Basel) 155, 194–204 (1968)

Collignon, J., Pryot, E.: La guanethidine a-t-elle une place dans le traitement d l'hypertension oculaire? Bull. Soc. belge Ophthal. 165, 344–349 (1973)

Crombie, A.L.: Adrenergic hypersensitization as a therapeutic tool in glaucoma. Trans. Ophthal. Soc. U.K. 94, 570–572 (1974)

Emmelin, N.: Supersensitivity following "pharmacological denervation", Pharmacol. Rev. 13, 17–37 (1961)

Etienne, R.: The non-myotical topical therapy of chemic glaucoma simplex. Amer. Med. Ass. Meeting, Section Ophthalmology (1973)

Garner, L.L., Johnstone, W.W., Balantine, E.J., Carroll, M.E.: Effect of 2% Levo-Rotary Epinephrine on the intraocular pressure of the glaucomatous eye. Arch. Ophthal. 62, 230–238 (1959)

Gloster, J.: Guanethidine and glaucoma. Trans. Ophthal. Soc. U.K. 94, 573–577 (1974)

Hampel, C.W.: The effect of denervation on the sensitivity to adrenaline of the smooth muscle in the nictitating membrane of the cat. Amer. J. Physiol. 111, 611–621 (1935)

Harris, L.S., Galin, M.A., Lerner, R.: The influence of Low-Dose L-Epinephrine on aqueous outflow facility. Ann. Ophthal. 2, 253–257 (1970)

Hendley, E., Eakins, K.: The mechanism of action of guanethidine on aqueous humour dynamics. J. Pharmacol. exp. Ther. 150, 393–397 (1965)

Küchle, H.J.: Zur lokalen Wirkung von guanethidine (Ismelin) auf das gesunde und glaukomkranke Auge. Klin. Mbl. Augenheilk. 139, 224–234 (1961)

Kutschera, E.: Klinische Erfahrungen mit Ismelin. Klin. Mbl. Augenheilk. 139, 234–241 (1961)

Merté, H.J., Toppel, L.: Guanethidine in der Glaukomtherapie. Albrecht v. Graefes Arch. Ophthal. 176, 30–42 (1968)

Mitchell, J.R., Oates, J.A.: Guanethidine and related agents. I. Mechanism of the selective blockade of adrenergic neurons and its antagonism by drugs. J. Pharmacol. exp. Ther. **172**, 100–107 (1970)

Nagasubramanian, S., Tripathi, R.C., Poinoosawny, D., Gloster, J.: Low concentration guanethidine and adrenaline therapy of glaucoma. Trans. Ophthal. Soc. U.K. **96**, 179–183 (1976)

Paterson, G.D., Paterson, G.: Drug therapy of glaucoma. Brit. J. Ophthal. **56**, 288–294 (1972)

Paterson, G.D., Paterson, G., Miller, S.H.J.: The non-myotic therapy of open angle glaucoma, in Albi Int. Glaucoma Symp. 343–352 (1974)

Romano, J.: Trial with guanethidine 5% and neutral adrenaline 1% in eyes with advanced glaucoma. Trans. Ophthal. Soc. U.K. **94**, 576–577 (1974)

Roth, J.A.: Guanethidine and adrenaline used in combination in chronic simple glaucoma. Brit. J. Ophthal. **57**, 507–510 (1973)

Sears, M.L.: The mechanism of action of adrenergic drugs in glaucoma. Invest. Ophthal. **5**, 115–119 (1966)

Stepanik, J.: Tonographische und differentialtonometrische Untersuchungen über die Wirkung von Ismelin-Augentropfen (Ciba) bei glaucoma simplex. Albrecht v. Graefes Arch. Ophthal. **164**, 6–9 (1961)

Tamura, T.: Effect of guanethidine on the vesiculated axon in the dilator muscle area of the rabbit iris. Jap. J. Ophthal. **17**, 140–146 (1973)

Trendelenburg, U.: Supersensitivity and subsensitivity to sympathomimetic amines. Pharmacol. Rev. **15**, 225–276 (1963)

Weekers, R., Pryot, E., Gustin, J.: Recent advances and future prospects in the medical treatment of ocular hypertension. Brit. J. Ophthal. **38**, 742–746 (1954)

Weekers, R., Delmarcelle, Y., Gustin, J.: Treatment of ocular hypertension by adrenaline and diverse sympathomimetic drugs. Amer. J. Ophthal. **40**, 666–672 (1955)

Weekers, R., Grieten, J., Collignon, J., Demaret, M.: Etude du mécanisme de l'hypotension oculaire provoquée par l'adrénaline. Docum. Ophthal. (Den Haag) **20**, 175–183 (1966)

CHAPTER VII

The combination of guanethidine 3% and adrenaline 0·5% in 1 eyedrop (GA) in glaucoma treatment

PH. F. J. HOYNG AND C. L. DAKE

SUMMARY   During a 7-month period 33 patients (20 with primary open-angle glaucoma and 13 with suspected glaucoma) were treated with guanethidine 3% and adrenaline 0·5% in 1 eyedrop twice daily. The previous therapy was discontinued and the aim of the trial was to treat the patients with GA alone. There was an average decrease in intraocular pressure of 10·8 mmHg or 37·5% for the whole group (including 5 patients with additional therapy). In eyes with an average IOP in a day-curve without medication equal to or higher than 28 mmHg we found a decrease in IOP of 44·6% or 14·4 mmHg, and in eyes with an average IOP without medication between 21 and 28 mmHg a decrease of 30·4% or 7·6 mmHg. With GA alone the IOP was 3·3 to 3·9 mmHg lower than on the previous therapy (P < 0·05); 46% of the eyes without additional therapy had all IOPs lower than 22 mmHg and 74% of the eyes had IOPs lower than 22 mmHg except 1 with a peak lower or equal to 25 mmHg 3 hours after application. This peak 3 hours after application indicates that GA has a biphasic action and was significant at the 0·5% level. Red eyes and slight ptosis were no problem for most patients. Patients found it very convenient to administer GA only twice daily.

During the last 10 years non-miotic therapy has taken a more important place in the treatment of glaucoma patients suspected of having glaucoma and primary open-angle glaucoma (POAG). One of the non-miotic preparations used is a combination of guanethidine and adrenaline. Stepanik (1961), Kutschera (1961), Küchle (1961), Oosterhuis (1962), and Bonomi and di Comite (1967) reported a fall in intraocular pressure (IOP) with guanethidine 10% alone in the treatment of patients with POAG. This fall was only temporary. Sears (1966) showed in studies on patients with Horner's syndrome 'that the outflow mechanism can be made supersensitive to topical epinephrine'. G. D. and G. Paterson (1972, 1974) pointed to the phenomenon of hypersensitivity of the receptor for sympathomimetic drugs during chemical denervation with guanethidine and to the necessity of applying adrenaline twice daily during the treatment with guanethidine. Long-term studies on guanethidine and adrenaline in patients with glaucoma have been done by Roth (1973), Ftienne (1973), Crombie (1974), Gloster (1974), Romano (1974, 1977), Nagasubramanian et al. (1976), and Jones et al. (1977) with good

results.

The aim of the trial reported here was to investigate the possibility of stopping all previous therapy of patients known to have POAG or suspected of having glaucoma, to treat them only with guanethidine 3% and adrenaline 0·5% (GA) in 1 eyedrop, and to investigate the proper dosage of GA. New patients with POAG or new glaucoma suspects were, if possible, treated only with GA. Thus we obtained an impression of the efficacy of GA alone and its effect in relation to previous therapy.

Patients and methods

Thirty-three patients (23 male and 10 female) with either POAG or suspected glaucoma were admitted to the trial. They were divided into 20 patients with POAG (33 eyes, 2 eyes having been previously operated on) and 13 glaucoma suspects (26 eyes). The mean age of the patients was 60 years (range 25 to 84 years), and treatment lasted for an average of 7 months (range 1 to 11 months).

Our criteria for diagnosing primary open-angle glaucoma were visual field defect and/or disc pathologically excavated and/or in a day-curve without medication 1 pressure higher than 36 mmHg, and with an open angle. Our criteria for glaucoma suspects were no visual field defect, normal disc, in the day-curve without medication at least 1 pressure higher than 25 mmHg and lower than 36 mmHg, and with an open angle. If a patient had one eye with glaucoma and the fellow eye showed only a raised IOP, both eyes were regarded as having POAG. These criteria are arbitrary. In our clinic we prefer to use the term glaucoma suspect instead of ocular hypertension.

Before the patients were admitted to the trial they were evaluated. Visual acuity and refraction were tested, biomicroscopy with the Haag-Streit slit lamp, and gonioscopy with the 3-mirror contact lens of Goldmann were undertaken, and visual fields were tested on a Tübingen perimeter. Patients were taken off treatment 1 week before the trial if they had been on sympathomimetics and carbonic anhydrase inhibitors and 48 hours beforehand if on miotics. A day-curve without medication was then made. The IOP was taken with a Goldmann applanation tonometer mounted on a Haag-Streit slit lamp at 9 a.m. and 12 noon (0 to 3 hours) and 3 p.m. and 5 p.m. (6 to 8 hours). The previous therapy which was stopped in these patients is shown in Table 1.

After a day-curve without medication all patients started with GA twice daily at an interval of 12 hours (at 9 a.m. and 9 p.m.). The day-curves were repeated after treatment for 1 week, 1 month, 3 months, and 7 months, and then medication with GA was stopped for 2 weeks, when the day-curve was repeated. GA was given after the first pressure reading in the day-curve. Thus the first reading (at zero) gave the IOP 12 hours after the last application. Additional therapy was given to patients in whom the IOP was not sufficiently lowered. Every month during the trial the patients were examined at our polyclinic for a short control period when we checked visual acuity, refraction, and IOP, and looked for side effects. Visual fields were controlled during our trial, and we particularly looked for changes in the early defects.

In the group with 20 patients with POAG 2 left the trial (1 patient died suddenly, and 1 left for personal reasons). Additional therapy in this group was needed in 4 patients. One patient needed acetazolamide once daily plus pilocarpine 2% 4 times daily. One (who died suddenly) needed acetazolamide once daily. One needed acetazolamide once daily and carbachol 1·5% 3 times daily. And 1 patient received only pilocarpine 2% twice daily. The rest of the group was controlled with GA twice daily only.

Table 1 *Previous therapy of 20 patients with POAG and 13 with suspected glaucoma*

20 patients with POAG (n = 33)	No. of eyes	13 glaucoma suspects (n = 26)	No. of eyes
Pilocarpine 2% 4 × d	14	Pilocarpine 1% 4 × d	4
Aceclidine 2% 4 × d	3	Pilocarpine 2% 4 × d	10
Aceclidine 2% 2 × d	2	Isoptocarpine 4 × d	4
Aceclidine 2% + adrenaline 1% 2 × d	5	Aceclidine 5 × d	2
Eserine 0·25% 4 × d	3	Eserine 0·25% 4 × d	2
Carbachol 1·5% 3 × d	2	Adrenaline borate 1 or 2 × d	10
Adrenaline borate 1% 2 × d	15	L-adrenaline bitartrate 2 × d	2
Ismelin 5%	3	Ismelin 5% 2 × d	2
Acetazolamide sustained release 1 × d	4	2 or 3 × 0·5 Acetazolamide	6
Acetazolamide 0·250 2 or 3 × d 0·5	4	None	4
None	5		

× d = times a day. Aceclidine = 3-acetoxyquinuclidine HCl.

In the group with suspected glaucoma 1 patient was taken off medication with GA because of transient serous maculopathy. She was known to have had maculopathy previously. One patient needed additional therapy with pilocarpine 1% twice daily. The rest of the group was controlled with GA twice a day only.

Our results were statistically evaluated by Student's *t* test.

Results

Fig. 1 and Table 2 show the combined results of all patients treated with GA for about 7 months. The average decrease in IOP for all patients (patients with additional therapy included) was 10·8 mmHg or 37·5%, with a reduction in fall of IOP to 7·4 mmHg or 26·7% after 3 hours. After 7 months' treatment the fall in IOP was still continuing and no adaptation was seen.

We have selected the eyes of patients who had no additional therapy in 2 groups. The first group with 22 eyes had an average IOP in a day-curve without medication higher than or equal to 28 mmHg. In the second group 25 eyes had an average IOP in a day-curve without medication between or equal to 21 and 28 mmHg (28 mmHg is about the median IOP of the averaged IOPs of the individual day-

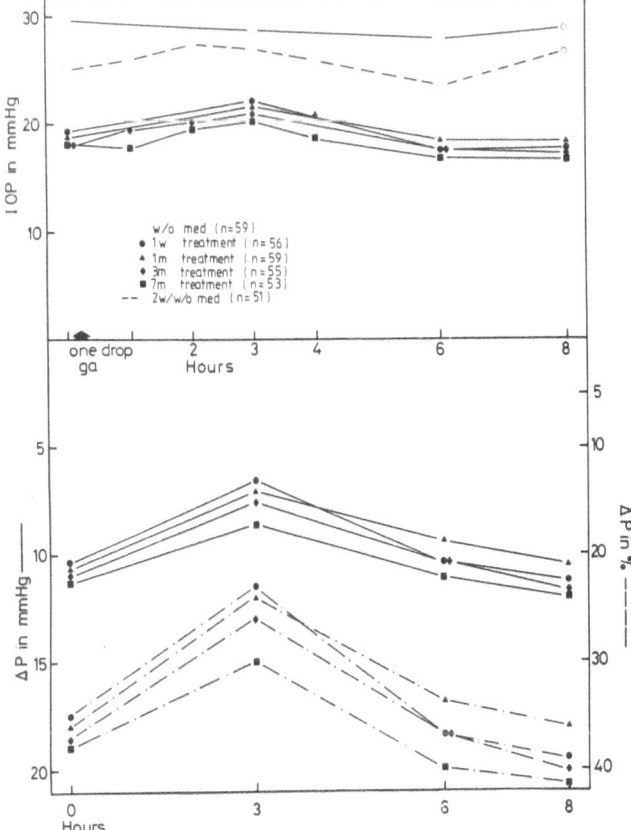

Fig. 1 Upper half: *Mean IOP day-curves of 33 patients with either POAG or suspected glaucoma during treatment (5 patients with additional therapy included).* Lower half: *ΔP in mmHg (solid line) and ΔP in percentages (dotted line)*

Table 2 *The results of treating 33 patients (59 eyes) with either POAG or suspected glaucoma (5 patients with additional therapy included), in mmHg ± standard error of mean*

	Hours			
	0	3	6	8
Mean IOP in mmHg without medication (n = 59)	29·5 ± 0·98	28·9 ± 0·90	27·9 ± 1·08	28·9 ± 1·15
Mean IOP in mmHg after 7 days' treatment (n = 56)	19·2 ± 0·69	22·3 ± 0·87	17·6 ± 0·69	17·7 ± 0·82
Mean IOP in mmHg after 1 month's treatment (n = 59)	18·9 ± 0·58	21·9 ± 0·67	18·5 ± 0·56	18·4 ± 0·63
Mean IOP in mmHg after 3 months' treatment (n = 55)	18·5 ± 0·51	21·4 ± 0·68	17·6 ± 0·57	17·3 ± 0·70
Mean IOP in mmHg after 7 months' treatment (n = 53)	18·3 ± 0·60	20·3 ± 0·59	16·8 ± 0·51	16·9 ± 0·52
Mean IOP in mmHg after 2 weeks without medication (n = 53)	25·0 ± 0·63	26·9 ± 0·81	23·7 ± 0·78	26·7 ± 0·98

± = standard error of mean.

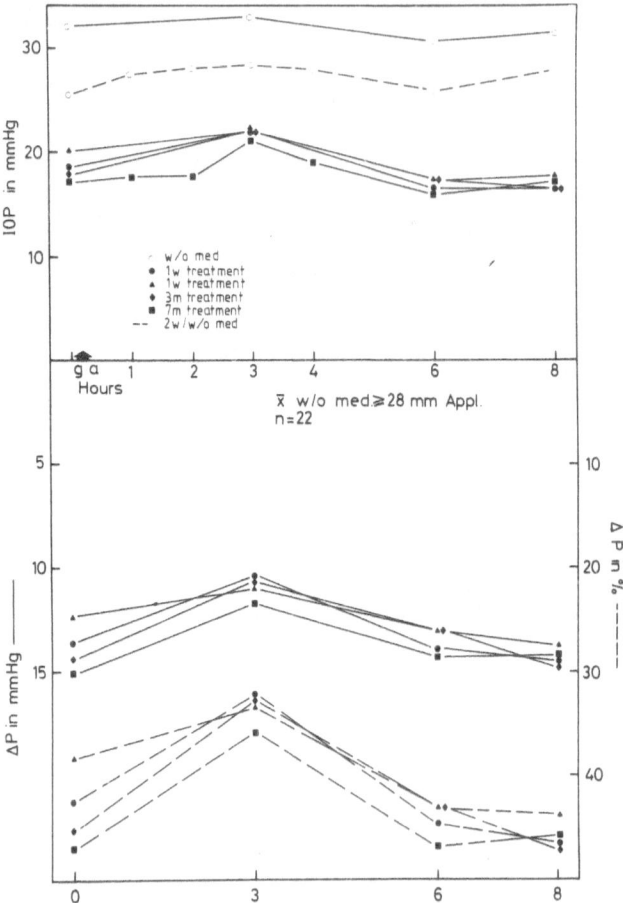

Fig. 2   Upper half: *Mean IOP day-curves of 22 eyes treated only with GA with an average IOP in the day-curve without medication equal to or higher than 28 mmHg. Lower half: ΔP in mmHg (solid line) and ΔP in percentages (dotted line)*

curves without medication). Figs 2 and 3 show the results.

There was a striking difference in percentage decrease of IOP. It was 44·6% for the eyes belonging to the group with the higher IOPs and 30·4% for the eyes with the lower IOPs. In Fig. 2 there is a fall in IOP from 31·7 mmHg (average of day-curves without medication) to 17·3 mmHg (average basal level with GA), and in Fig. 3 there is a fall from 24·8 mmHg (average of the day-curves without medication) to 17·2 mmHg (average basal level with GA).

It is interesting to note that, whatever the initial

mean IOP was without medication, 24·8 or 31·7 mmHg, there seemed to be a decrease in IOP to a basal limit of 17 mmHg. We do not know the reason for this phenomenon.

The results in the individual patients are shown in Table 3. Twenty-three eyes were well controlled and all had an IOP lower than or equal to 21 mmHg. Twenty-three eyes were controlled and had all IOPs lower than 22 mmHg except at least one peak pressure 3 hours after application in one of the day-curves during treatment. In 14 eyes this peak pressure was lower than or equal to 25 mmHg, and in 9 eyes there were peak pressures between 25 and

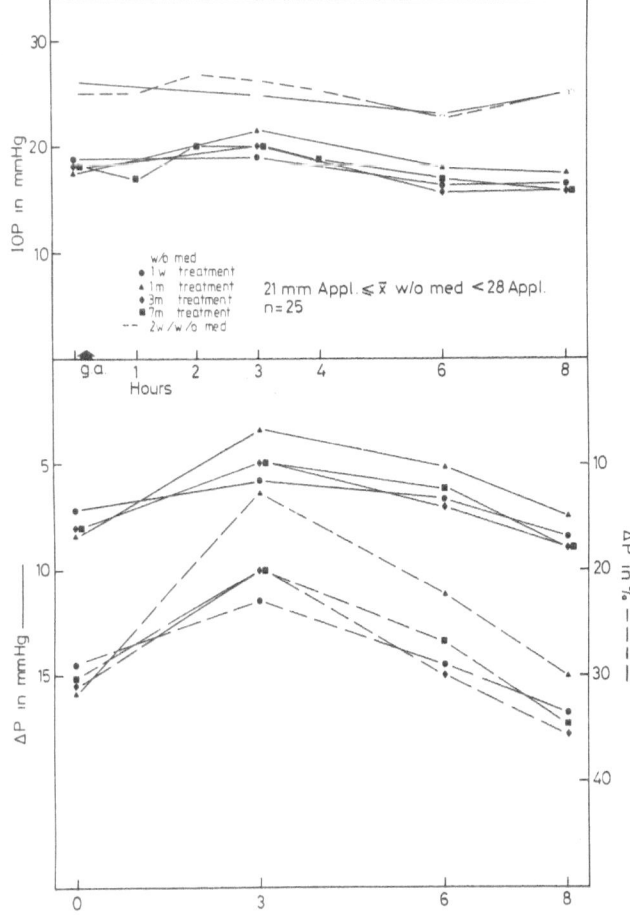

Fig. 3 Upper half: *Mean IOP day-curves of 25 eyes treated only with GA with an average IOP in the day-curve without medication equal to or greater than 21 mmHg and lower than 28 mmHg. The lower half shows ΔP in mmHg (solid line) and ΔP in percentages (dotted line)*

30 mmHg. Nine eyes were not controlled but had a good fall in IOP. In 2 patients (4 eyes) there was no response at all.

Among the patients who were treated with GA alone 46% of eyes had all IOPs lower than 22 mmHg during and after the 7-month period, and 74% had all IOPs lower than 22 mmHg with now and then a peak pressure in a day-curve but not higher than 25 mmHg. The patients who needed additional medication were included in the not well controlled group but with a good fall in IOP. The POAG patient with no response at all, had acetazolamide

and pilocarpine 2% 4 times daily as additional therapy. The glaucoma suspect with no response had an initial good response on GA but tachyphylaxis developed.

We compared the results of 12 POAG patients and 9 glaucoma suspects, who were treated with GA alone, with the control level they showed on the previous therapy. The results are shown in Table 4. It indicates that in 18 patients (33 eyes) there was a lower controlling IOP level with GA alone than with previous therapy (3·3 to 3·92 mmHg; P < 0·05). In 1 POAG patient the level with GA alone

Table 3 *Number of eyes controlled by GA*

	POAG (n=33)	Glaucoma suspects (n=26)	Total (n=59)
Well controlled	12	11	23
Controlled	14	9	23
Uncontrolled but with decrease in IOP	5	4	9
No response	2	2	4

Table 4 *Mean individual differences in IOP of 21 patients (38 eyes) treated with GA alone with respect to their mean individual IOP on previous treatment; n = number of eyes. For POAG patients the mean number of measurements during previous medication is 12·5 and for glaucoma suspects 14*

	12 POAG	9 Glaucoma suspects
Mean lower IOP level in mmHg with GA	-3·92 (n=15)	-3·3 (n=18)
Equal mean IOP level with GA	(n=2)	—
Mean higher IOP level in mmHg with GA	+0·8 (n=3)	—

was the same and 2 POAG patients (3 eyes) had a higher pressure with GA alone (0·8 mmHg).

The number of measurements taken during the previous therapy were 12·5 (range 5 to 25) for the POAG patients and 14 (range 7 to 24) for glaucoma suspects. These were measurements taken during examinations at the polyclinic and not when day-curves were done.

SIDE EFFECTS
Only 2 patients found the drops unpleasant and had cosmetic objections. One of these had severe redness of the eye with chemosis and severe ptosis (more than 3 mm). The other had only moderate hyperae-mia of the conjunctiva bulbi et tarsi. Fifteen patients with slight redness and 5 with moderate redness of the eyes had no objections to continuing treatment because of this. Transient or slight ptosis (1 to 2 mm) was found in 7 patients and moderate ptosis (2 to 3 mm) in 2. In 2 patients there was evidence of transient keratoepitheliopathy, but this did not lead to interruption of medication. Six patients had reading problems during the first hours after application. In 4 patients (4 eyes) early visual field defects disappeared and in 1 patient with an absolute visual field defect the defect progressed in spite of an excellent response on IOP. Tachyphylaxis was seen in 1 glaucoma suspect after

3 months' treatment. One patient showed serous maculopathy in 1 eye after 1 month's treatment, which disappeared 3 months later after GA was discontinued. She was known to have maculopathy previously. It was not regarded as a side effect but as progression of the underlying maculopathy.

Discussion

Guanethidine is thought to remove the stored noradrenaline in the granulated vesicles of the sympathetic nerve endings, to block the re-uptake, and to cause a depletion of noradrenaline at the nerve ending. As a result hypersensitivity for sympathomimetics develops at the receptor side. Since the Patersons started to use adrenaline in combination with guanethidine many studies on this subject have been done. Until now GA has not yet gained an important place in the treatment of glaucoma. This is partly owing to the side effects and partly owing to unfamiliarity with GA.

We have carried out this detailed study because we believe that more knowledge about its less well known properties was needed. We consider that we have in GA a potential mixture for lowering IOP, though there is some reduction of the effect on IOP 3 hours after application. This reduction is about 3·5 mmHg for the whole group (P < 0·005). A detailed analysis of this peak effect with GA 3 hours after application will be published elsewhere. The biphasic response during GA treatment has not been previously reported.

In comparison with previous therapy, all patients (except 2 with red eyes) found it pleasanter to administer the drops only twice daily. Hyperaemia of the conjunctivae and slight or moderate ptosis was acceptable to most patients. Visual acuity did not change except in 1 patient known to have progressing cataract. Refraction showed a slight increase in hypermetropia of $\frac{1}{4}$ to $\frac{3}{4}$ dioptre in 7 patients. After GA was stopped this disappeared. Relaxation of the ciliary muscle may be the cause of it. Reading problems during the first few hours after application of GA disappeared with $\frac{1}{4}$ dioptre stronger presbyopia correction for reading. We do not know whether this is due to widening of the pupil or a slight increase in hypermetropia. Reading problems were mainly in patients aged between 40 and 55. Patients who complained of dark vision with miotics lost these symptoms with GA. Widening of the pupil during the first hours after application was frequently seen.

Summarising, we find that with GA, despite red eyes and slight ptosis, we have an effective conservative treatment for patients with suspected glaucoma and POAG. Younger patients, who had many problems with miotics, respond particularly well on GA. Operations may be delayed in patients who were not responding to previous therapy. Combinations with other conservative treatments are possible.

We gratefully acknowledge the skilful assistance of Mrs J. Loeb, who performed the tonometry, and Mr A. Blijleve, who made the drawings. We thank ZYMA for providing us with Z-15000 PD-70 during the trial.

References

Bonomi, L., di Comite, P. (1967). Outflow facility after guanethidine sulfate administration. *Archives of Ophthalmology*, **78**, 337–340.

Crombie, A. L. (1974). Adrenergic hypertensitisation as a therapeutic tool in glaucoma. *Transactions of the Ophthalmological Societies of the United Kingdom*, **94**, 570–572.

Etienne, R. (1973). The non-miotic topical therapy of chronic glaucoma simplex. American Medical Association Meeting, Section of Ophthalmology.

Gloster, J. (1974). Guanethidine and glaucoma. *Transactions of the Ophthalmological Societies of the United Kingdom*, **94**, 573–577.

Jones, D. E. P., Norton, D. A., and Davies, D. J. G. (1977). Low dosage combined adrenaline-guanethidine formulations in the management of chronic simple glaucoma. *Transactions of the Ophthalmological Societies of the United Kingdom*, **97**, 192–196.

Küchle, H. J. (1961). Zur lokalen Wirkung von Guanethidine (Ismelin) auf das gesunde und glaukomkranke Auge. *Klinische, Monatsblätter für Augenheilkunde*, **139**, 224–234.

Kutschera, F. (1961). Klinische Erfahrungen mit Ismelin. *Klinische Monatsblätter für Augenheilkunde*, **139**, 234–241.

Nagasubramanian, S., Tripathi, R. C., Poinoosawny, D., and Gloster, J. (1976). Low concentration guanethidine and adrenaline therapy in glaucoma. *Transactions of the Ophthalmological Societies of the United Kingdom*, **96**, 179–183.

Oosterhuis, J. A. (1962). Guanethidine (Ismelin) in ophthalmology. *Archives of Ophthalmology*, **67**, 592–599.

Paterson, G. D., and Paterson, G. (1972). Drug therapy of glaucoma. *British Journal of Ophthalmology*, **56**, 288–294.

Paterson, G. D., Paterson, G., and Miller, S. H. J. (1974). The non-miotic therapy of open angle glaucoma, in *Albi International Glaucoma Symposium*, 343–352.

Romano, J. (1974). Trial with guanethidine 5% and neutral adrenaline 1% in eyes with advanced glaucoma. *Transactions of the Ophthalmological Societies of the United Kingdom*, **94**, 576–577.

Romano, J. (1977). Use of guanethidine 5 per cent and adrenaline 1 per cent in the treatment of severe open angle glaucoma. *Transactions of the Ophthalmological Societies of the United Kingdom*, **97**, 196–202.

Roth, J. A. (1973). Guanethidine and adrenaline used in combination in chronic simple glaucoma. *British Journal of Ophthalmology*, **57**, 507–510.

Sears, M. J. (1966). The mechanism of action of adrenergic drugs in glaucoma. *Investigative Ophthalmology*, **5**, 115–119.

Stepanik, J. (1961). Tonographische und differentialtonometrische Untersuchungen über die Wirkung von Ismelin-Augentropfen (Ciba) bei glaucoma simplex. *Albrecht von Graefes Archiv für klinische und experimentelle Ophthalmologie*, **164**, 6–9.

CHAPTER VIII

VERIFICATION OF THE BIPHASIC RESPONSE IN INTRAOCULAR PRESSURE DURING TREATMENT OF GLAUCOMA PATIENTS WITH 3% GUANETHIDINE AND 0.5% ADRENALINE

ABSTRACT

In a long-term study with 3% guanethidine and 0.5% adrenaline in one eye drop (GA) the combined results of patients with primary open angle glaucoma (POAG) and glaucoma suspects showed a biphasic response in intraocular pressure (IOP). The hypertensive phase peaked 3 hrs after administration (at noon) and reached a maximum of 3.5 mm Hg (p < 0.005) above the hypotensive phase. It is reported in the literature that during office hours untreated glaucoma patients show a peak near noon, suggesting that the initial increase in IOP may be the normal IOP pattern.

When the data of untreated patients with POAG and glaucoma suspects were separated, an increase in IOP around noon in the first group and a decrease around noon in the glaucoma .suspects was found. However, during GA-treatment both groups showed a hypertensive response at noon (3 hrs). In addition, the highest IOP's in daycurves were timed during and without GA. It was shown that during GA there was a shift in the incidence of the highest IOP's towards noon (from 8.3% to 73.2% for patients with suspected glaucoma and from 32% to 63.6% for those with POAG).

It was therefore concluded that GA induces a characteristic biphasic IOP pattern in patients with POAG as well as in glaucoma suspects. Also, glaucoma suspects may have higher peak pressures more frequently than POAG patients. Furthermore, the study showed that during office hours untreated glaucoma suspects have daycurves with higher pressures in the morning while patients with POAG have higher pressures near noon.

INTRODUCTION

A biphasic response in the behaviour of intraocular pressure (IOP) has been reported in normal rabbit eyes after noradrenaline (Langham & Palewitz, 1977) and adrenaline (Langham & Krieglstein, 1976). Sympathetically denervated rabbit eyes showed a similar biphasic response of IOP after adrenaline (Lamble, 1974) and noradrenaline (Unger & Hammond, 1977; Waitzman & Woods, 1979). The hypertensive response could be blocked with phenoxybenzamine in normal rabbit eyes (Langham & Krieglstein, 1976), and in denervated rabbit eyes (Unger & Hammond, 1977; Waitzman & Woods, 1979) indicating that alphareceptors mediated the initial rise in IOP.

A biphasic response of IOP has not been reported after adrenaline and noradrenaline in the human eye. However, in a clinical trial on patients with primary open angle glaucoma (POAG) and suspected glaucoma treated with 3% guanethidine and 0.5% adrenaline combined in one eyedrop (GA) twice

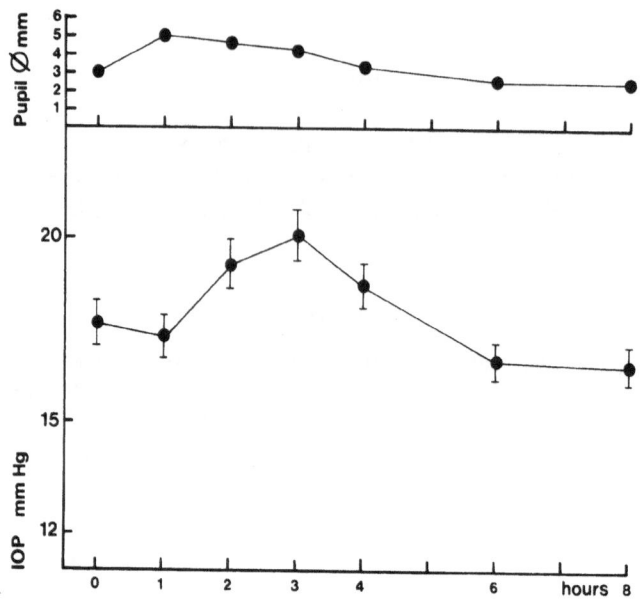

Fig. 1. Mean daycurves of intraocular pressure (IOP) and pupil size of fifteen patients with primary open angle glaucoma (POAG) and eleven glaucoma suspects together at seven months of treatment with guanethidine and adrenaline (standard error of the mean between bars).

Table 1. Mean intra-ocular pressure (IOP) ± standard error of the mean (SEM) in mm Hg and the mean pupil size ± SEM in mm of fifteen patients with primary open angle glaucoma (POAG; 24 eyes) and eleven glaucoma suspects (22 eyes) together at seven months of treatment with guanethidine and adrenaline.

Hours after adm. of GA	0	1	2	3	4	6	8
Mean IOP ± SEM in mm Hg.	17.7 0.59	17.3 0.55	19.3 0.66	20.1 0.57	18.7 0.62	16.7 0.43	16.6 0.50
Mean pupil diameter ± SEM in mm.	3.01 0.15	5.02 0.21	4.16 0.23	4.16 0.18	3.38 0.23	2.57 0.10	2.54 0.10

daily, a biphasic response was found in the pattern of the IOP daycurves (Hoyng & Dake, 1979) (Fig. 1, Table 1). During the first hours following repeated administration of GA the IOP increased by 2.8 mm Hg ($p < 0.005$) and at noon (3 h) IOP peaked at 3.5 mm Hg ($p < 0.005$) above the hypotensive phase. The hypotensive phase was quantified by taking average pressure readings during treatment at 0,6 and 8 hours. A similar biphasic response in the IOP after guanethidine and adrenaline was reported by Jones et al. (1979) and Urner-Bloch et al. (1980). The significance of the hypertensive response during the first hours after repeated administration of GA may be questionable, since the literature indicates that untreated glaucoma patients may show a peak at noon in daycurves taken during office hours. This could mean that the peak 3 hours after repeated administration of GA simply coincides with the normal IOP pattern in the daycurves of glaucoma patients. Therefore, a further analysis of this peak is needed.

MATERIALS AND METHODS

Out of a group consisting of 20 POAG patients and 13 glaucoma suspects treated with GA twice daily, those patients that were treated with GA alone, were selected. Fifteen POAG patients (24 eyes) and eleven glaucoma suspects (22 eyes) were then treated for a 7-month period with GA exclusively.

A patient was regarded as having POAG if the average IOP in a daycurve without medication was over 22 mm Hg, with either a visual field defect or a pathologically excavated optic disc or both, and with an open angle.

A patient was suspected of having glaucoma if the average IOP in a daycurve without treatment was over 22 mm Hg, with a normal visual field and optic disc, with no IOP over 36 mm Hg and with an open angle. If one eye had glaucoma and the fellow eye showed only an elevated IOP, then both eyes were regarded as having POAG.

After stopping all previous therapy for at least 48 hours, an IOP daycurve was made and the patients started on GA twice daily at 9.00 a.m. and 9.00 p.m. The daycurves with therapy were repeated after 1 week, 1 month, 3 months and 7 months of treatment. An IOP daycurve consisted of at least four pressure readings taken during office hours, while an IOP curve over 24 hours with pressure readings also during the night was defined as a diurnal IOP curve. GA was applied after the first pressure reading of the daycurve (9.00 a.m.). Therefore, the first reading at zero time represents the IOP 12 hours after the last application of GA. It has already been mentioned that the hypotensive phase was quantified by taking average pressure readings during GA treatment at 0, 6 and 8 hours. Further relevant details are published elsewhere (Hoyng et al., 1979).

The shapes of the mean IOP daycurves with and without treatment for the 15 patients with established glaucoma were then compared with the corresponding mean IOP daycurves of the 11 patients suspected of having glaucoma. Further, the time of the highest IOP out of the readings at 0, 3, 6 and 8 hours in the daycurves of the individual patients during and without treatment was noted. If the highest IOP was noted at two or more time points, the value was divided in equal parts. The incidence of the highest IOP's in the daycurves of the POAG patients with and without treatment was compared with that for the glaucoma suspects.

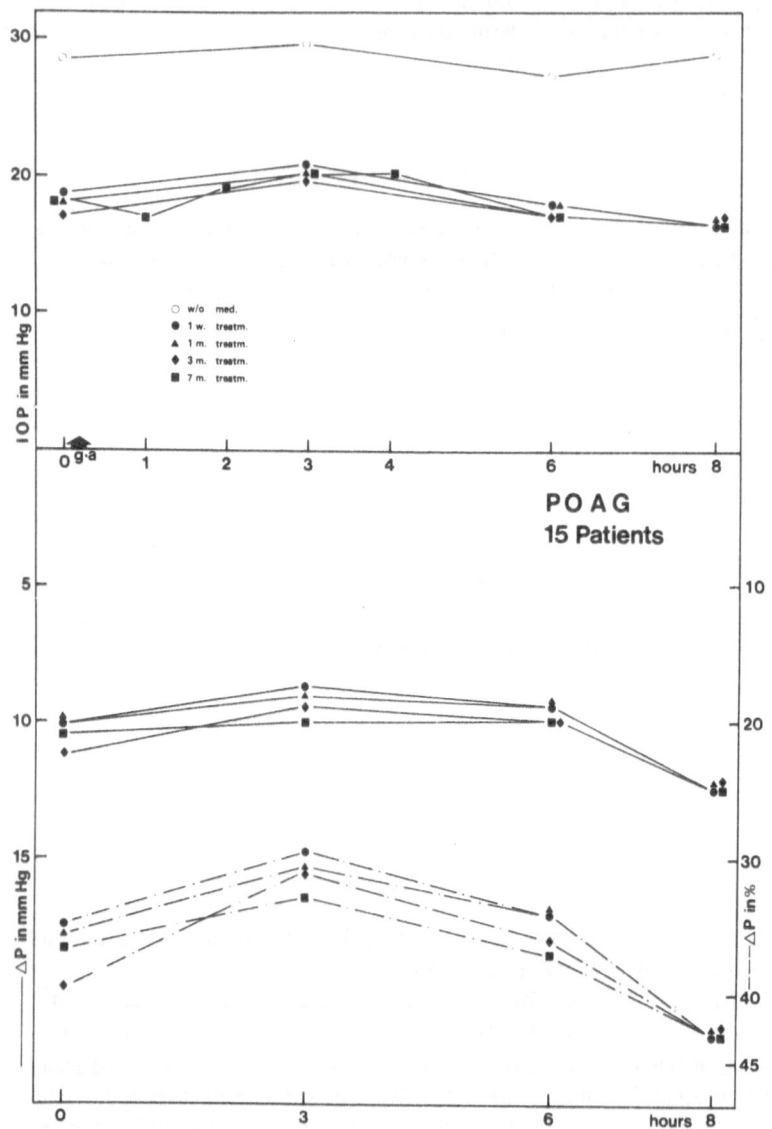

Fig. 2a. *Upper half:* Mean IOP in daycurves of fifteen patients with POAG (24 eyes) with and without treatment.
Lower half: Δp (IOP untreated − IOP treated) in mm Hg (solid line) and in percent (dotted line).

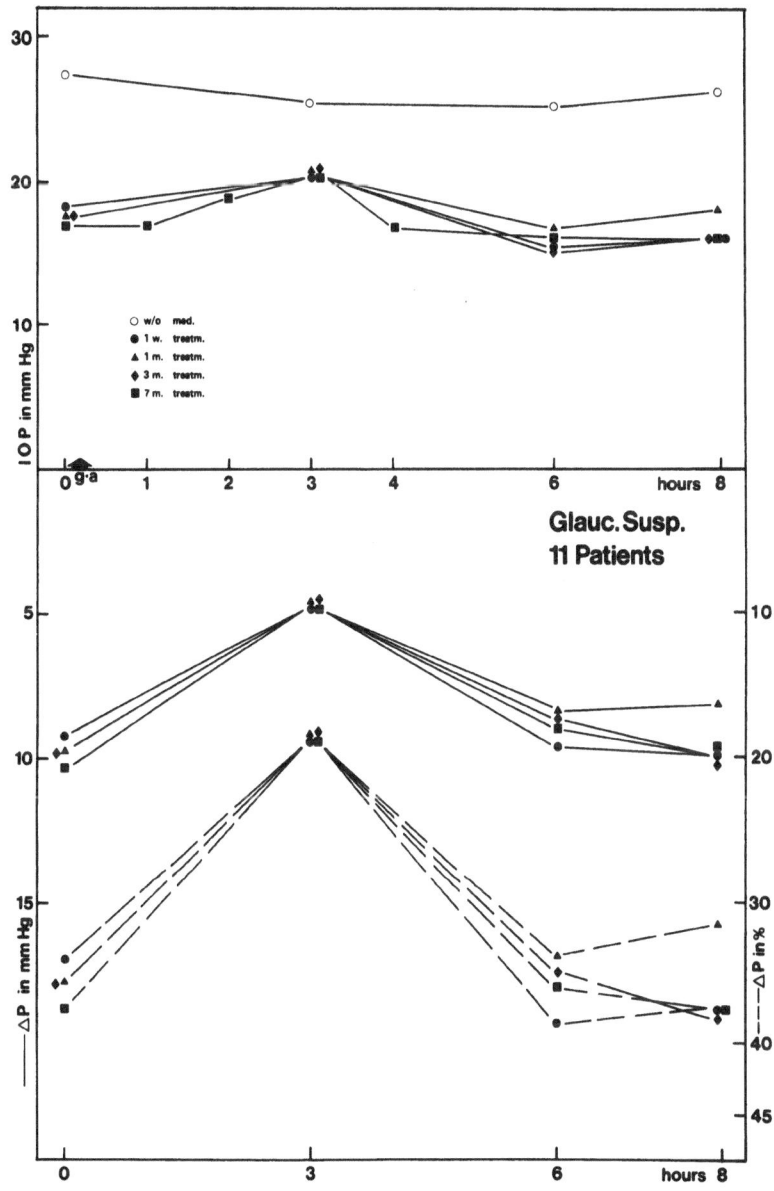

Fig. 2b. *Upper half:* Mean IOP daycurves of eleven patients with suspected glaucoma (22 eyes) with and without treatment.
Lower half: △p in mm Hg (solid line) and in percent (dotted line).

Finally, the shape of the mean daycurves and the incidence of the highest IOP's in a randomized group consisting of 60 patients with POAG (111 eyes, average age 63.7 years) and 37 patients with suspected glaucoma (74 eyes, average 65.7 years), all without medication, were compared. The results were statistically evaluated using the t-test for pairs.

RESULTS

POAG patients

Figure 2a and Table 2 show the results in 15 patients with POAG (24 eyes) treated with GA alone. In the lower half of the figure a 38% fall in IOP in the hypotensive phase is expressed. In the hypertensive phase, 3 hours after administration of GA, the fall in IOP is reduced to 31%. The mean IOP in the hypotensive phase is 17.5 mm Hg, which is increased by 2.8 mm Hg to 20.3 mm Hg at noon during the hypertensive phase ($p < 0.005$). In the mean daycurve of untreated POAG patients there is an increase in IOP of 1.2 mm Hg ($p > 0.05$) at noon compared to the pressure readings at zero time.

Table 2. Mean IOP ± SEM in mm Hg of fifteen patients with POAG (24 eyes) with and without 3% guanethidine and 0.5% adrenaline (GA).

Hours after application	0	3	6	8
Mean IOP ± SEM in mm Hg without medication of POAG patients	28.4 ±1.4	29.6 ±1.5	27.4 ±1.2	29.0 ±1.6
Mean IOP ± SEM in mm Hg during 7 months treatment with GA for POAG patients	18.1 ±0.37	20.3 ±0.44	17.7 ±0.36	16.6 ±0.33
Δp in mm Hg during 7 months with GA for POAG patients	10.3	9.3	9.7	12.4
Δp in percentages during 7 months treatment with GA for POAG patients	36.3	31.4	35.4	42.8

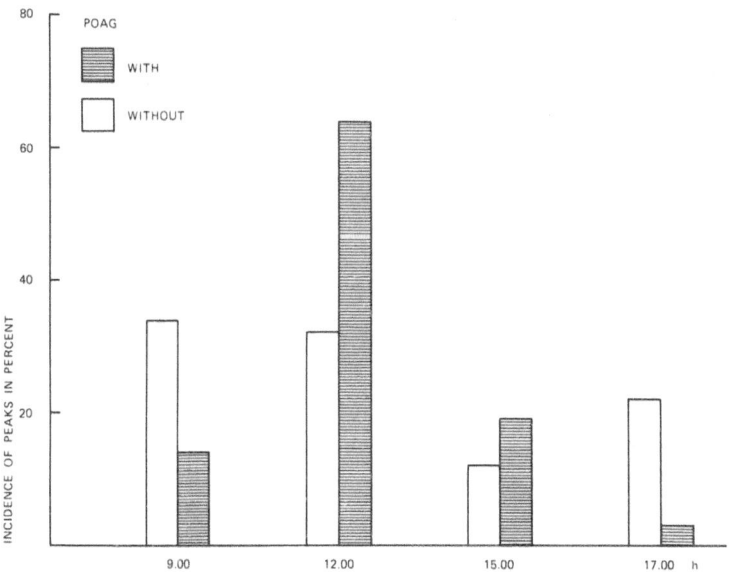

Fig. 3a. Incidence of the highest IOP's in percent of fifteen patients with POAG with and without GA-treatment.

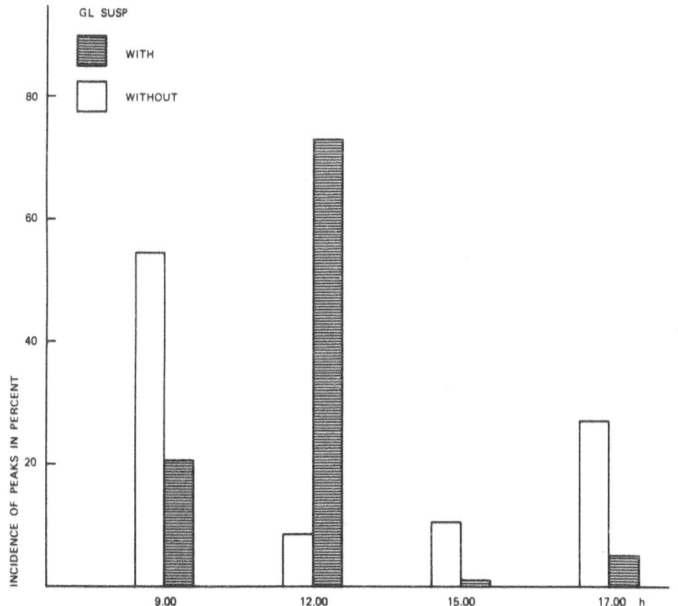

Fig. 3b. Incidence of the highest IOP's in percent of eleven patients with suspected glaucoma with and without GA-treatment.

Table 3. Mean IOP ± SEM in mm Hg of eleven patients with suspected glaucoma (22 eyes) with and without GA-treatment.

Hours after application	0	3	6	8
Mean IOP ± SEM in mm Hg without medication of glaucoma susp.	27.3 ±1.04	25.2 ±0.9	25.0 ±1.09	26.0 ±1.03
Mean IOP ± SEM in mm Hg during 7 months with GA for glaucoma suspects	17.5 ±0.39	20.5 ±0.47	16.0 ±0.32	16.6 ±0.35
ΔP in mm Hg during 7 months with GA for glaucoma suspects	9.8	4.7	9.0	9.4
ΔP in percentages during 7 months treatment with GA for glaucoma suspects	35.7	18.8	36.0	36.2

Table 4. Incidence of the highest IOP's in percent in daycurves of fifteen patients with POAG and eleven patients with suspected glaucoma with and without GA-treatment.

TIME		9.00	12.00	15.00	17.00
POAG	WITHOUT MEDICATION	34	32	12	22
	WITH GA	14.1	63.6	19.0	3.3
GL. SUSP.	WITHOUT MEDICATION	54.1	8.3	10.4	27.1
	WITH GA	20.7	73.2	1.1	5.0

Figure 3a and Table 4 show the incidence of the highest IOP's in the day-curves of 15 POAG patients during and without treatment. The incidence of the highest IOP's in daycurves without medication is hardly different at 9.00 a.m. and 12.00 a.m. (34% and 32%, respectively), but during treatment the incidence of the highest IOP's decreases from 34% to 14.1% at 9.00 am. and increases from 32% to 63.6% at noon.

84

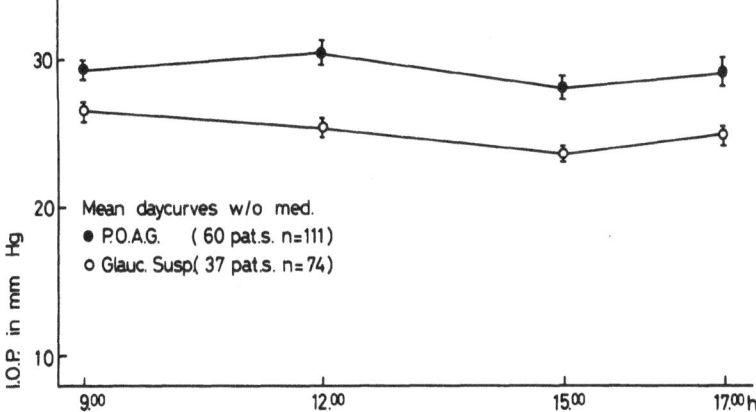

Fig. 4. Mean daycurves ± SEM in mm Hg of sixty patients with POAG (111 eyes) and of thirtyseven patients with suspected glaucoma (74 eyes) without medication.

Table 5. Mean IOP ± SEM in mm Hg of sixty patients with POAG (111 eyes) and thirty-seven patients with suspected glaucoma (74 eyes), all without treatment.

Time	9.00	12.00	15.00	17.00
Mean I.O.P. ▲ S.E.M. in mm Hg of 60 P.O.A.G. pat.(n=111)	29,32 ▲ 0,71	30,37 ▲ 0,68	28,03 ▲ 0,73	29,17 ▲ 0,84
Mean I.O.P. ▲ S.E.M. in mm Hg of 37 Glauc.Susp.(n=74)	26,52 ▲ 0,60	25,45 ▲ 0,57	23,58 ▲ 0,53	24,73 ▲ 0,60

Figure 4 and Table 5 show the mean IOP daycurve without medication for 60 patients with POAG (111 eyes) selected at random. The shape of the mean IOP daycurve shows an increase in IOP at noon with respect to the values at 9.00 a.m. (1.05 mm Hg, $p < 0.01$). The incidence of the highest IOP's in these patients, figure 5 and table 6, is the highest at noon with 43.9%.

Glaucoma suspects

The results for the 11 glaucoma suspects, comprising 22 eyes treated with GA alone, are presented in figure 2b and table 3. In the lower half of the figure a 36% fall in IOP in the hypotensive phase is expressed. This fall in IOP is reduced to 19% in the hypertensive response. The mean IOP during the hypotensive response is 16.7 mm Hg, increasing by 3.8 mm Hg to 20.5 mm Hg at noon during the hypertensive phase ($p < 0.005$). In the mean daycurve of the untreated glaucoma suspects the IOP is decreased by 2.1 mm Hg at noon compared to the first pressure readings ($p < 0.05$).

Figure 3b and table 4 show the incidence of the highest IOP's in the day-curves of 11 patients with suspected glaucoma during and without treat-ment. In the daycurves without medication the incidence of the highest

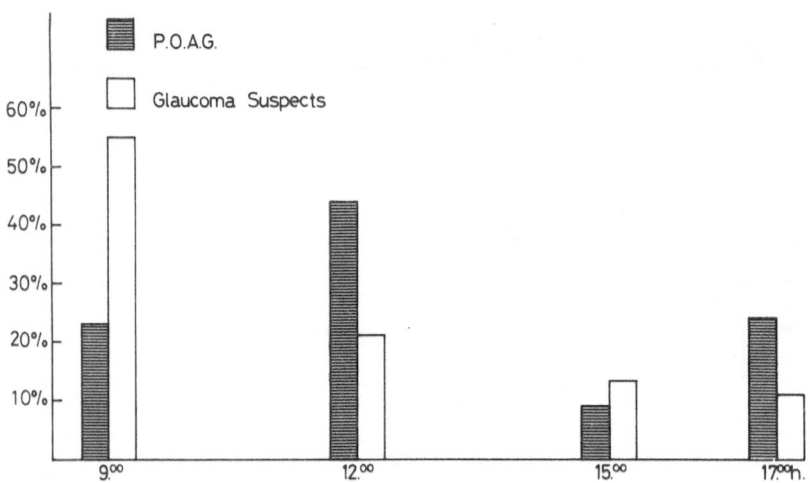

Fig. 5. Incidence of the highest IOP's in percent in daycurves of sixty patients with POAG and thirty-seven patients with suspected glaucoma without medication.

Table 6. Incidence of the highest IOP's in percent in daycurves of sixty patients with POAG and thirty-seven patients with suspected glaucoma without medication.

TIME		9.00	12.00	15.00	17.00
POAG	111 Eyes	23,2%	43,9%	9,2%	23,7%
Glauc. Susp.	74 Eyes	54,7%	20,9%	13,5%	10,8%

IOP's is 54.1% at 9.00 a.m. and 8.3% at noon. However, during treatment the incidence of the highest IOP's decreases from 54.1% to 20.7% at 9.00 a.m. and increases from 8.3% to 73.2% at noon.

Figure 4 and table 5 show the mean IOP daycurve without medication for 37 patients with suspected glaucoma (74 eyes). The shape of the mean IOP daycurve shows decrease in IOP at noon compared to the values at 9.00 a.m. (1.07 mm Hg, p < 0.005). The incidence of the highest IOP's in these patients, figure 5 and table 6, is the highest at 9.00 a.m. with 54.7%.

DISCUSSION

With IOP daycurves, taken during office hours in untreated glaucoma patients, Bitran (1968) reported the highest IOP's at 9.00 a.m. and 12.00 a.m. In diurnal IOP curves Drance (1960) and Leydhecker (1973) recorded the highest IOP's in 60% of glaucoma patients during non-office hours, but during office hours the data reported by Drance show a higher incidence of peaks near noon. Leydhecker found a second peak near noon (first peak before rising between 6.00 and 8.00 a.m.).

The results reported here for 60 patients with POAG and 37 patients with suspected glaucoma show a significant difference in shape of the mean IOP daycurves without treatment. While the mean IOP increases at noon with respect to the values at 9.00 a.m. in POAG patients, it decreases at noon for the patients with suspected glaucoma (fig. 4). The difference in pattern of the mean IOP curves is enhanced by the difference between these two groups of patients in incidence of the highest IOP's (fig. 5). It indicates that in daycurves taken during office hours and consisting of four measurements (9.00 and 12.00 a.m., and 3.00 and 5.00 p.m.) patients with POAG tend to have their highest IOP's near noon (43.9%) and patients with suspected glaucoma at 9.00 a.m. (54.7%).

The shape of the mean IOP daycurves of these patients and the incidence of peaks correlate with the shape of the mean IOP daycurves and incidence of peaks in the 15 patients with POAG and 11 with suspected glaucoma before they were treated with GA (fig. 2a, b upper half).

During treatment the data at zero time and at 3 hours in table 2 and 3 indicate that there is a slight reduction in the fall of IOP in POAG patients and a much larger reduction in the fall of IOP in glaucoma suspects at noon (3 hrs). This might suggest that there is a basic difference in the IOP pattern between POAG patients and glaucoma suspects on GA treatment. The upper half of figure 2a shows the mean daycurves with and without treatment for the POAG patients. At noon, both curves shown an increase in IOP compared to the pressure readings at zero time: 2.2 mm Hg ($p < 0.05$) and 1.2 mm Hg ($p > 0.05$), respectively. This results in an absolute difference between the two peaks of only 1 mm Hg.

At noon, the mean daycurve of the untreated glaucoma suspects shows a decrease in IOP of 2.1 mm Hg ($p < 0.05$) compared to the pressure readings at zero time (fig. 2b), while during treatment there is an increase in IOP of 3.0 mm Hg ($p < 0.05$). Hence the absolute difference between the noon values for treated and untreated eyes is now 5.1 mm Hg. The levelling of the peak to 1 mm Hg in POAG patients and the increase to 5.1 mm Hg in glaucoma suspects are expressed in the lower half of fig. 2a and 2b, in which Δp (IOP untreated − IOP treated) is plotted on the ordinate.

It was already mentioned that the reduction in IOP in the hypotensive phase is hardly different between patients with POAG and glaucoma patients (38% and 36%, respectively), and that the measurements at 3 hours in the hypertensive phase show a greater difference, viz. 31% for POAG patients and 19% for glaucoma suspects. But, the mean IOP during treatment with GA significantly increases at noon in both groups of patients, resulting in a similar biphasic response of the mean IOP daycurves (upper half of fig. 2a and 2b). In addition, timing of the highest IOP's in the daycurves of the individual patients during and without GA reveals that during GA treatment there is a shift in the incidence of the highest IOP's towards noon in patients with suspected glaucoma as well as in patients with POAG (from 8.3% to 73.2% for glaucoma suspects and from 32% to 63.6% for POAG patients, fig. 3a, 3b and table 4).

Although in POAG patients the patterns of the mean IOP daycurves with and without treatment are not significantly different, the shift in the incidences of highest IOP's (fig. 3a, 3b) clearly shows that GA induces a biphasic pattern in both group of patients, which is more pronounced in glaucoma suspects than in POAG patients.

During treatment of GA peaks of 5 mm Hg or more were found in 45% of the IOP daycurves of patients with suspected glaucoma and in 26% of the IOP daycurves of patients with POAG near noon. Hence, treatment with GA may result in a biphasic response of the IOP in both groups of patients.

Preliminary results of investigations on the origin of the biphasic response of IOP reveals, that after GA the dilation of the pupil has no influence on the behaviour of IOP. Tonographic analysis reveal a 36% increase in aqueous humour production in the hypertensive phase ($p < 0.02$). Outflow facility was not significantly different. This subject will be reported in a subsequent paper.

REFERENCES

Bitran, D. Evaluacion de la curve de tension diaria. *Arch. Chil. Oftal.* 25: *32-39* (1968). Abstract Zbl. ges. *Ophthal.* 103: *125* (1970).

Drance, S.M. The significance of the diurnal tension in variations in normal and glaucomatous eyes. *Arch. Ophthal.* 64: *494-501* (1960).

Hoyng, Ph. F. J. & Dake, C. L. The combination of guanethidine 3% and adrenaline 0.5% in one eye drop (g-a) in glaucoma treatment. *Brit. J. Ophthal.* 63: *56-62* (1979).

Jones, D. E. P., Norton, D. A. & Davies, D. J. G. Control of glaucoma by reduced dosage guanethidine-adrenaline formulations. *Brit. J. Ophthal.* 63: *813-816* (1979).

Lamble, J. W. The effect of topically applied guanethidine sulphate on the pupil and tension responses of the rabbit eye to (-) adrenaline bitartrate. *Exp. Eye Res.* 19: *79-89* (1974).

Langham, M. E. & Krieglstein, G. K. The biphasic intra-ocular pressures response of rabbits to epinephrine. *Invest. Ophthal.* 15: *119-127* (1976).

Langham, M.E. & Palewicz, K. The pupillary, the intra-ocular pressure and the vaso-motor responses to nor-adrenaline in rabbits. *J. Physiol.* 267: *339-355* (1977).

Leydhecker, W. Glaukom. Ein Handbuch. Zweite völlig neubearbeitete Auflage. Seite 410-415. Springer Verlag, Berlin – Heidelberg – New York, (1973).

Unger, W. G. & Hammond, B. R. Nor-adrenaline – induced inflammation in the sym-pathectomised rabbit eye. *IRCS Med. Sci.* 5: *563* (1977).

Urner-Bloch, U., Bucheli, J., Eltz, H., Gloor, J.B. & Aeschlimann, J. Clinical trials of various glaucoma drugs acting on the adrenergic system. *Klin. Mbl. Augenheilk.* 176: *555-558* (1980).

Waitzman, M. B. & Woods, W. D. Effects of prostaglandins, norepinephrine on intra-ocular pressure and pupil size in rabbits following cervical ganglionectomy. *Invest. Ophthal.* 18: *52-60* (1979).

CHAPTER IX

PUPIL BEHAVIOUR AND RESPONSE OF INTRAOCULAR PRESSURE

PH. F. J. HOYNG & C. L. DAKE

ABSTRACT

In the study reported here, the relation between the dilatation of the pupil and the course of intracoular pressure (IOP) is examined in open angle glaucoma patients and in glaucoma suspects after topical administration of the combination of guanethidine 3% and adrenaline 0.5% in one eye drop (GA). By treating one eye with GA and leaving the fellow eye untreated on the same day, there was a symmetrical response of IOP, independent of the mydriasis in the treated eyes. It leads to the conclusion that the mydriatic response has no influence on the course of IOP. The physiological explanation for the symmetrical course of IOP in both treated and untreated fellow eyes seems to be a mediation by the bloodstream of GA to the eye which was left untreated.

INTRODUCTION

A significant biphasic response of intraocular pressure (IOP) was reported in primary open angle glaucoma patients (POAG) and in patients with suspected glaucoma (SG) during a long term treatment with the combination guanethidine 3% and adrenaline 0.5% in one eye drop (GA) (Hoyng & Dake, 1979). During the first few hours after repeated administration of GA the IOP increases. The hypertensive response coincides with the mydraitic response and peaks 3.5 mm Hg over the hypotensive phase (p < 0.005).

After an initial fall a transient increase in IOP two hours post-GA was reported in a single dose response study (Jones, Norton & Davies, 1979), showing an IOP day curve for GA similar to those we obtained (Hoyng, Dake & Greve, 1977). Jones and co-workers suggested that 'the transient increase in IOP might be the consequence of pupillary dilation in some patients'.

The aim of the trial reported here was to investigate the relation between the mydriatic response and the behaviour of IOP during a long term treatment with GA in patients with open angle glaucoma.

PATIENTS AND METHODS

Out of 33 patients with either POAG or SG who were admitted to a trial with GA twice daily (at 9 a.m. and 9 p.m.) during five months, five POAG patients and seven SG patients were selected at random.

Before they were admitted to the long term study gonioscopy was performed and the angle has been examined with and without mydriasis. Only patients with proven open angles were admitted to the study. All patients except one were treated in both eyes with GA alone. One

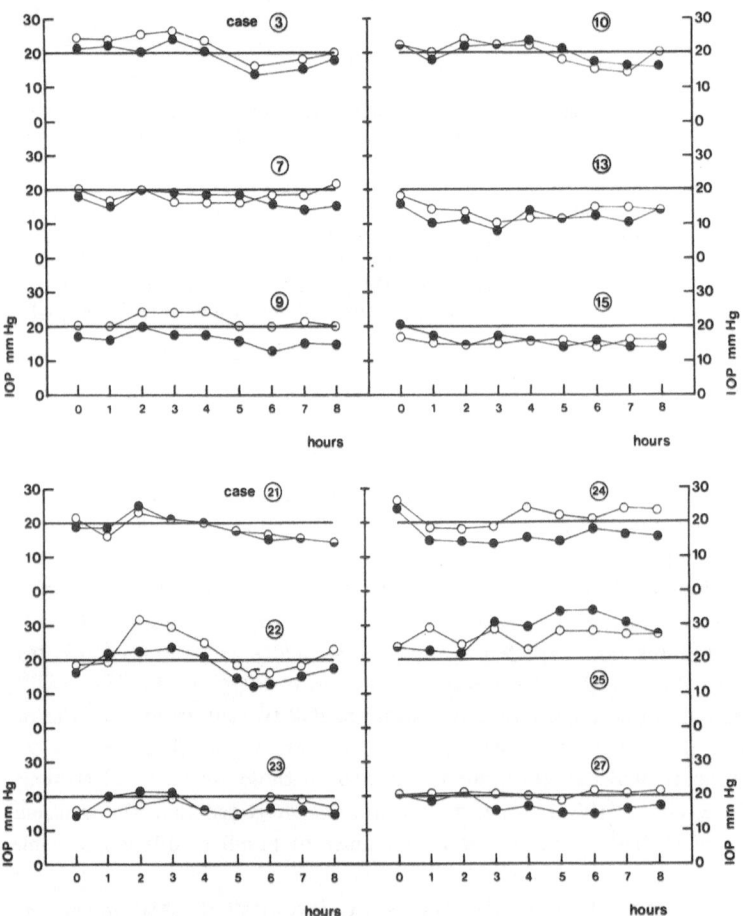

Fig. 1-2. The individual IOP daycurves in mm Hg. Closed circle indicates the GA treated eye, open circle the untreated fellow eye on the same day.

92

POAG patient required an additional Diamox sustet (sustained release) at 9 a.m. The patients were asked to make their last application of GA at 5 p.m. The next day they visited the clinic and pupil size and IOP were examined every hour from 9 a.m. till 5 p.m. The first measurement at 9 a.m. (zero time) thus presents the data 16 hours after the last administration. After the first measurements, one drop of GA was administered only to the eye with the lower IOP. The fellow eye with the higher IOP during GA treatment, remained untreated on the same day, and the measurements taken give the data between 16 and 24 hours after the last administration of GA, i.e. at 5 p.m. the day before. In the treated eyes with the lower IOP the measurements were taken between 0 and 8 hours after GA application. All patients continued medication on both eyes after they had finished the trial.

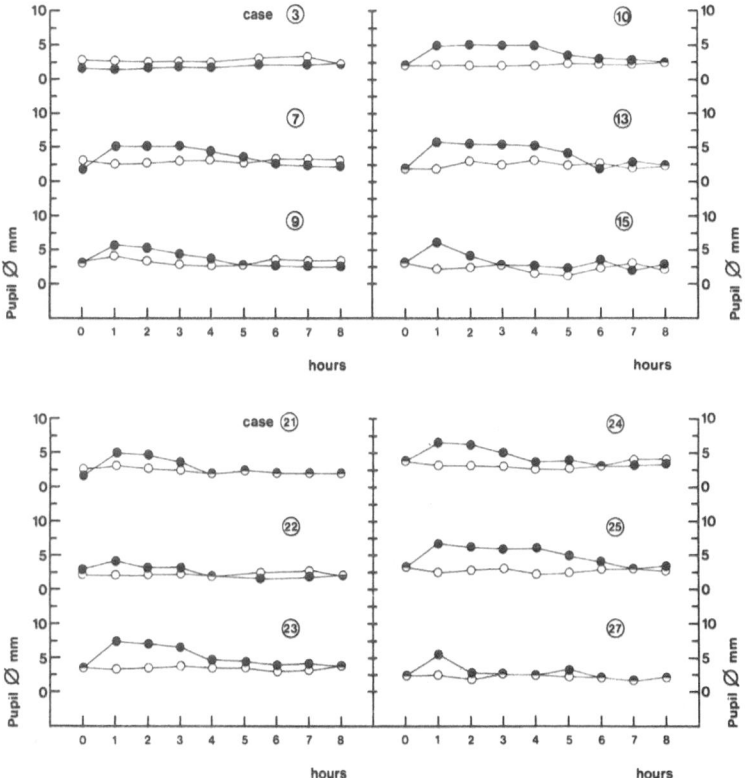

Fig. 3-4. The individual behaviour of the pupil diameter in mm. Closed circle indicates the GA treated eye, open circle the untreated fellow eye on the same day.

The pupil diameter was measured under standardized light conditions with a calibrated ocular on the Goldmann perimeter. The IOP was taken with the Goldmann applanation tonometer mounted on a Haag-Streit slit-lamp.

RESULTS

Figures 1 and 2 present the individual daycurves of the 12 treated eyes (closed circles) and untreated fellow eyes (open circles) on the same day.

Figures 3 and 4 present the individual behaviour of the corresponding pupil sizes. The symmetry in the course of the individual IOP daycurves of treated and untreated fellow eyes show a striking contrast with asymmetry in the behaviour of the corresponding individual pupil sizes. Since, barring case 3, the pupils of the eyes treated with GA dilated during the first few hours following administration. The diameter of the pupils in the untreated fellow eyes remained unchanged.

Figure 5, and tables 1 and 2 present the data of the average IOP daycurve and the average pupil size of the 12 treated eyes and untreated fellow eyes. It sets off even more the difference in behaviour of the pupil and the symmetrical course of the IOP in the treated and untreated eyes on the same day.

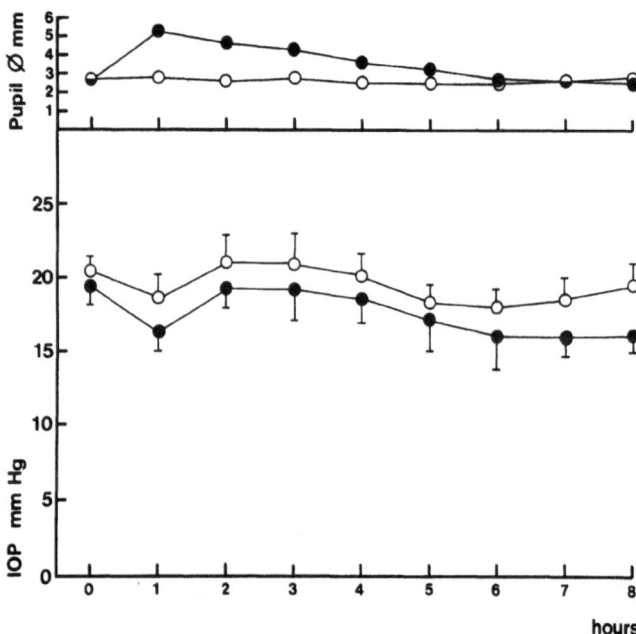

Fig. 5. The mean IOP daycurve ± standard error of the mean (SEM) in mm Hg and the mean course of the pupil diameter in mm Hg. Closed circles indicates GA treated eyes, open circles the untreated fellow eyes on the same day.

Table 1. The mean IOP ± standard error of the mean (SEM) in mm Hg and the mean course of the pupil ± SEM in mm of the treated eyes with lower IOP's. At zero time one drop GA was applied. Asterisk indicates zero time 16 hours after the last administration of GA.

Hours after administration of GA	0	1	2	3	4	5	6	7	8
Mean IOP ± SEM in mm Hg after 5 months of treatment	19.3* ±0.93	17.3 ±0.97	19.1 ±1.03	18.9 ±1.67	18.5 ±1.25	17.2 ±1.68	16.3 ±1.68	16.0 ±1.33	16.3 ±1.06
Mean pupil sizes ± SEM in mm after 5 months of treatment	2.54* ±0.19	5.33 ±0.44	4.67 ±0.45	4.30 ±0.41	3.60 ±0.39	3.30 ±0.29	2.70 ±0.19	2.67 ±0.18	2.45 ±0.17

Table 2. The mean IOP ± SEM in mmHg and the mean course of the pupil size in mm ± SEM of the fellow eyes which were left untreated on the same day.

Hours after administration of GA	16	17	18	19	20	21	22	23	24
Mean IOP ± SEM in mm Hg after 5 months of treatment	20.3 ±0.89	18.6 ±1.20	20.9 ±1.42	20.8 ±1.67	19.8 ±1.20	18.3 ±1.13	18.2 ±1.11	18.6 ±1.10	19.4 ±1.12
Mean pupil sizes ± SEM in mm after 5 months of treatment	2.67 ±0.17	2.67 ±0.20	2.54 ±0.17	2.62 ±0.14	2.42 ±0.16	2.54 ±0.13	2.67 ±0.15	2.71 ±0.21	2.63 ±0.21

COMMENT

Elevation of IOP with cycloplegic or sympathomimetic drugs is enigmatic in gonioscopically open angle glaucoma patients. Kronfeld (Kronfeld, McGarry & Smith, 1943) showed a slight increase in IOP with homatropine and paredrine in 15 eyes of POAG patients. Galin (1961) reported a positive response of IOP to cyclopentolate with an accompanying decrease in outflow facility, in nine patients with open angle glaucoma. Harris (1969) found a cycloplegic-induced elevation of IOP in 23% of a population with proven open angle glaucoma compared to 2% in a normal population. In the same trial phenylephrine 10% failed to produce a significant increase in IOP. Lee (1958) reported an occasional prolonged and significant increase in IOP in open angle glaucoma patients following topical administration of adrenaline 1% or phenylephrine 10%. Hill (1968) showed an increase in IOP in 20% of gonioscopically open angle glaucoma patients following mydriasis with phenylephrine 10%. Recently Mapstone (1978) reported on a provocative test with pilocarpine 2% and phenylephrine 10% in 68 open angle glaucoma patients (119 eyes). He observed the same response compared to normal eyes in 22% only. In the trial reported here, a combination of guanethidine 3% and adrenaline 0.5% was used. Guanethidine is thought to remove the stored noradrenaline from the granulated vesicles in the axoplasma of the sympathetic nerve endings. It further prevents the re-uptake of noradrenaline resulting in a depletion at the distal sympathetic nerve endings. Hypersensitivity for sympathomimetic drugs develops at the sympathetic receptor site (Mitchell & Oates, 1970). The response of the pupil and IOP to topical adrenaline is therefore far more potent in pharmacologically denervated eyes, compared to normal eyes (Holland & Wei, 1973). During a 7 months' study with GA we observed a mydriatic response greater than 2 mm in 50% of the patients, The mydriatic response coincides with the hypertensive response, while the hypotensive phase coincides with the slowing down of the mydriatic response. It was suggested that the transient rise of IOP was related to the pupillary dilation (Jones et al, 1977). In the pooled data of the patients in this study the biphasic IOP response was not significant. The individual and pooled data of the pupil sizes and the corresponding IOP's of twelve treated and twelve untreated eyes show that the dilatation of the pupil has no influence on the course of IOP and that if there is an increase in IOP this is not restricted to the GA treated eyes.

This study shows that there is no evidence of a mydriasis-induced effect on IOP behaviour following the first few hours after administration of GA. The question may arise why the continuing fall in IOP was not restricted to the treated eyes, why the untreated fellow eyes showed almost the same course of IOP and why no difference in direct effect on IOP was found regardless of whether the eye was treated or left untreated. We took great care to prevent drug contamination by the tonometer tip. Furthermore both eyes were pharmacologically denervated for a long period, so that reflex action via sympathetic fibres to the untreated fellow eye seems improbable. After topical treatment with one eye drop of guanethidine 10% Wolff (1969), using the fluorometer method of Weekers-Delmarcelle, showed a direct inhibition in the rate of aqueous production in the treated eyes and the same effect in the untreated fellow eyes after an interval of 10 minutes. The effects on the aqueous rate and the interval of 10 minutes might suggest drug mediation by the blood stream to the untreated fellow eye. This study shows that after a long period on continuous treatment with GA there is no difference in the course of IOP of both eyes, when one eye is treated and the fellow eye left untreated on the same day. Hence the physiological explanation for the symmetrical course of IOP seems to be GA mediation by the blood stream to the untreated fellow eye. Further it shows that after administration of GA the dilation of the pupil has no influence on the course of IOP, provided the angle was open.

ACKNOWLEDGEMENTS

We gratefully acknowledge the skillful assistance of Mrs. J. Loeb, who performed the tonometry, and Mr. A. Blijleve, who made the drawings. We thank DISPERSA for providing us with SUPREXON 3-0.5 (GA) during trial.

REFERENCES

Galin, M. A. The mydriasis provocative test. *Arch. Ophthal.* 66: *353-355* (1961).

Harris, L. S. Cycloplegic-induced intraocular pressure evaluations. A study of normal and open glaucomatous eyes. *Arch. Ophthal.* 79: *242-246* (1969).

Hill, K. What's the angle on mydriasis? *Arch. Ophthal.* 79: *804* (1968).

Holland, M.G. & Wei, C. P. Epinephrine dose-response characteristics of glaucomatous human eyes following chemical sympathectomy with 6-hydroxydopamine. *Ann. Ophthal.* 5/6: *633-640* (1973).

Hoyng, Ph. F. J., Dake, C. L. & Greve, E. L. A double-blind short-term trial of guanethidine 3% and adrenaline 0.5% combined in one eye-drop. *Graefes Arch. Ophthal.* 203: *73-80* (1977).

Hoyng, Ph. F. J. & Dake, C. L. The combination of guanethidine 3% and adrenaline 0.5% in one eye-drop (G-A) in glaucoma treatment. *Brit. J. Ophthal.* 63: *56-62* (1979).

Jones, D. E. P. Norton, D. A. & Davies, D. J. G. Control of glaucoma by reduced dosage guanethidine-adrenaline formulation. *Brit. J. Ophthal.* 63: *813-816* (1979).

Kronfeld, P., McGarry, H. I. & Smith, H. E. The effect of mydriatics upon the intraocular pressure in socalled primary open angle glaucoma. *Amer. J. Ophthal.* 26: *245-252* (1943).

Lee, P. F. The influence of epinephrine and phenylephrine in intraocular pressure. *Arch. Ophthal.* 60: *863-867* (1958).

Mapstone, R. Mechanisms in open angle glaucoma. *Brit. J. Ophthal.* 62: *257-282* (1978).

Mitchell, J. R. & Oates, J. A. Guanethidine and related agents. I. Mechanisms of the selective blockade of adrenergic neurons and its antagonism by drugs. *J. Pharmacol. Exp. Ther.* 172: *100-107* (1970).

Wolff, M. Wirkung von Guanethidine auf die Blutkammerwasserschranke. *Ber. dtsch. ophthal. Ges.* 70: *551-554* (1969).

CHAPTER X

The Aqueous Humor Dynamics and the Biphasic Response in Intraocular Pressure Induced by Guanethidine and Adrenaline in the Glaucomatous Eye

Ph.F.J. Hoyng and C.L. Dake

Abstract. Continuous administration of guanethidine (3%) and adrenaline (0.5%) in one eyedrop (GA) induced a biphasic response of intraocular pressure (IOP). In ten patients with primary open angle and seven glaucoma suspects treated with (GA) twice daily during a 7 month period, tonography, and tonometry were performed and the pupil diameter measured 3 and 8 h post-GA. The combined data of both groups in the hypertensive phase, showed an IOP increase of 2.8 mm Hg ($P < 0.05$), an unchanged coefficient of the outflow, dilated pupil (1.73 mm) ($P < 0.005$) and a 36% increase of aqueous humor production ($P < 0.02$). The specific biphasic course of IOP during treatment with GA seems to be caused by fluctuations in aqueous humor production. The increase in aqueous rate during the hypertensive phase could be related to secondary (rebound) vasodilation in the ciliary body and/or to a transient disruption of the blood-aqueous barrier induced by release of prostaglandins.

Introduction

In the treatment of glaucoma patients with one eyedrop of combined guanethidine (3%) and adrenaline (0.5) administered twice daily, a biphasic response of intraocular pressure (IOP) was found (Hoyng and Dake 1979) (Figs. 1 and 2). During the first hours following administration IOP increased by 2.8 mm Hg ($P < 0.005$) and peaked by 3.5 mm Hg ($P < 0.005$) over the hypotensive phase. The hypotensive phase was quantified by taking the average IOP readings at 0, 6 and 8 h during treatment. If, in patients who were treated in both eyes with GA one eye was then treated with GA, and the fellow eye left untreated, a symmetrical response of IOP was found regardless of the mydriasis in the treated eye (Hoyng and Dake, in preparation, 1980). Hence, it was concluded that the hypertensive response of IOP was not related to a decrease in outflow facility due to dilation of the pupil. The aim of this trial was to investigate aqueous humor dynamics during the hypertensive and hypotensive phases.

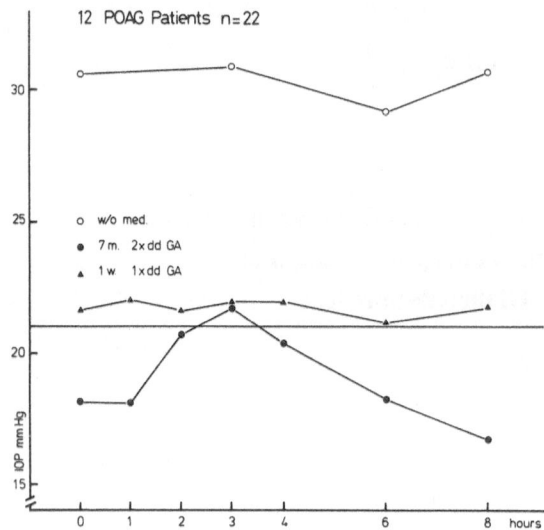

Fig. 1. Mean intraocular pressure (IOP) day curves of 12 patients with primary open angle glaucoma (POAG) after 7 months of twice-daily (2dd) guanethidine + adrenaline (GA) (measurements 0–8 h after GA) and after 1 week of once-daily GA (measurements 16–24 h after GA), and in the absence of therapy. The day curve with GA 2 dd reveals the biphasic IOP response

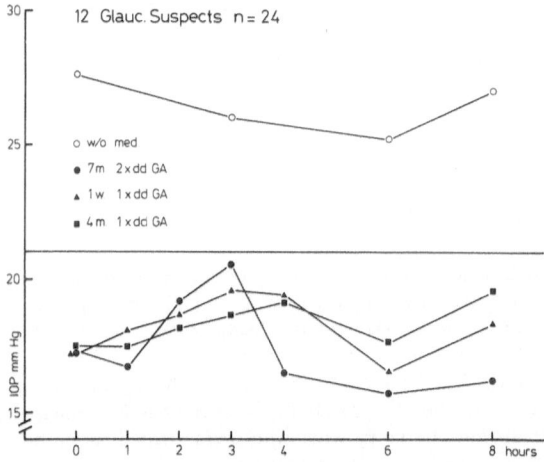

Fig. 2. Mean intraocular pressure (IOP) day curves of 12 glaucoma suspects after 7 months (7 m) of twice-daily (2 dd) guanethidine + adrenaline (GA) (measurements 0–8 h after GA) and after 1 week (1 w) and 4 months (4 m) of once-daily (1 dd) GA (measurements 16–24 h after GA), and in the absence of therapy. The day curve with GA 2 dd reveals the biphasic IOP response

100

Table 1. The mean Po in mm Hg±SEM, the mean coefficient (C) of outflow in µl/min/mm±SEM and the aqueous humour production (F) in µl/min ±SEM of ten primary open angle glaucoma (POAG) patients ($N=15$) and seven glaucoma suspects (SG) ($N=14$) apart and together

Hours after GA administration	POAG + SG		POAG		SG	
	3 h	8 h	3 h	8 h	3 h	8 h
Po in mm Hg± SEM	19.9 ±0.77[a]	17.1 ±0.85	20.0 ±0.93	17.3 ±1.31	19.8 ±1.33[b]	16.8 ±0.99
C µl/min/mm Hg± SEM	0.161 ±0.011	0.162 ±0.007	0.139 ±0.016	0.143 ±0.008	0.190 ±0.017	0.191 ±0.009
F µl/min ±SEM	1.49 ±0.12[a]	1.10 ±0.11	1.34 ±0.13	0.97 ±0.14	1.69 ±0.21	1.27 ±0.18
Pupil diameter in mm ±SEM	4.35 ±0.29[c]	2.62 ±0.13	4.20 ±0.36[c]	2.60 ±0.20	4.54 ±0.49[c]	2.63 ±0.18

[a] $P<0.05$
[b] $P<0.01$
[c] $P<0.005$

Materials and Methods

The patients and methods were similar to the comparative tonographic study of Hoyng and Dake (in preparation, 1980). Over a 7-month period ten patients with primary open angle glaucoma (15 eyes) and seven patients with suspected glaucoma (14 eyes) were treated with GA twice daily (9 a.m. and 9 p.m.). At the end of the 7-month period tonography was performed 3 and 8 h after application of GA with an interval of at least 2 days and no more than 1 week. At the same time, the pupil diameter was measured with the calibrated ocular on the Goldmann perimeter under standardized conditions.

The tonography was always performed by the same investigator to eliminate undesirable fluctuations. Applanation tonometry, followed by tonography, was first done on the right eye and, after a 15-min interval, on the left eye.

The coefficient of outflow was calculated according to the modification of Moses et al. (1968) of the Friedenwald tables. If necessary, corrections for scleral rigidity were made. The aqueous humor production was calculated from the formula, $F=C$ $(P_o\text{-}P_e)$, the applanation tonometry, taken prior to the tonography, being taken as P_o, while episcleral venous pressure was assumed to be 10 mm Hg. IOP was taken with a Goldmann applanation tonometer and the tonography was performed with a Müller electronic Schiøtz tonograph connected to an Esterline-Angus recorder. The data were statistically evaluated using the paired t-test. (Table 1).

Results

The results are shown in Fig. 3 and Table 1. In patients with primary open angle glaucoma there was an increase in IOP, the outflow facility was unchanged, and the aqueous humor production was increased at 3 h post-GA. Similar

101

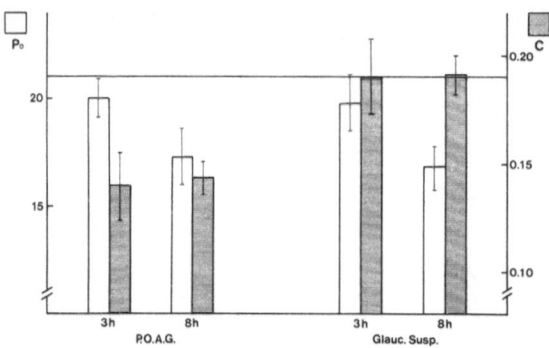

Fig. 3. The mean P_0 in mm Hg±SEM and the mean coefficient of outflow (C) in µl/min/mm Hg±SEM taken at 3 and 8 h after application of guanethidine + adrenaline (GA)

results were found in the patients with suspected glaucoma. The pooled data of the patients with primary open angle glaucoma and suspected glaucoma during the hypertensive phase showed an increase in IOP of 2.8 mm Hg ($P < 0.05$), an unchanged coefficient of outflow, an increased aqueous humor production of 36% ($P < 0.02$), and a dilation of the pupil of 1.73 mm ($P < 0.005$), as compared to the hypotensive phase.

Discussion

The fall in IOP after application of adrenaline is either due to inhibition of the formation of aqueous, to an increase in outflow facility, or to both and adrenaline also induces a transient dilation of the pupil. Pharmacological denervation of the ocular sympathetic system can be induced by several drugs, e.g., guanethidine, which is known to increase membrane permeability of the sympathetic nerve endings, leading to the release of noradrenaline (NA) stored in the granulated vesicles. Furthermore, guanethidine blocks the reuptake of NA, results in depletion in the distal sympathetic nerve endings, and, supersensitivity to catecholamines develops at the receptor site. Holland and Wei (1973) found, after pharmacological denervation with 6-hydroxydopamine in glaucoma patients, a supersensitivity to catecholamines in the adrenergic receptors, which mediate aqueous production and the pupil diameter. In addition Hoyng and Dake (in preparation, 1980) showed, after pharmacological denervation with guanethidine in glaucoma patients, a supersensitivity to adrenaline in the mechanisms that mediate outflow facility.

The biphasic response of IOP in GA treatment requires an explanation. The investigations of Langham and Krieglstein (1976) and Langham and Palewicz (1977) in rabbits suggested a fluctuation in outflow resistance. Langham and Krieglstein (1976) showed a biphasic response of IOP after repeated administration of adrenaline (1%). Furthermore, the hypertensive response in rabbits could be blocked with phenoxybenzamine, an α-adrenergic blocking agent, after IV or topical administration. This could indicate that the adrenaline-induced hypertensive response in rabbits, was due to α-adrenergic stimulation. In addition, pretreatment with the β-adrenergic blocking agent propranolol, had no influence on the hypertensive response. After repeated administration, Langham and Palewicz (1977) found a similar biphasic response of IOP with NA (4%). They showed that in rabbits the hypertensive and hypotensive response with NA was related to an increase and decrease of outflow resistance, respectively. It was postulated that the increase in outflow resistance in the hypertensive phase was due to a vasoconstriction of the epi- and intrascleral vessels collecting the aqueous humor.

Another explanation for the fluctuations in outflow facility is also possible. Van Alphen (1976) found that after β-adrenergic stimulation there was a relaxation of the ciliary muscle. A decrease in outflow facility could therefore be caused by inhibition of the pull in the scleral spur after GA administration. However, the impression was formed from this study, that, in man, after GA administration the biphasic IOP response was not related to fluctuations in outflow facility but to fluctuations in the formation of the aqueous humor. This was based on the observation that the increase in IOP was independent of the dilatation of the pupil. If one eye was treated with GA, and the fellow eye was left untreated on the same day, a similiar IOP response was found in both, while the treated eye alone showed dilation of the pupil. It could indicate that a decrease in outflow facility caused by dilation of the pupil was improbable (Hoyng and Dake, in preparation, 1980). Moreover, it was clearly shown in this tonographic study, that the hypertensive response was due to an increase in aqueous humor production, indicating that the ciliary processes mediate the biphasic effect of GA on IOP. Several mechanisms could therefore be responsible:

1) After GA administration there is not only a transient initial vasoconstriction of the conjunctival vessels, but also of the vessels of the ciliary processes which could lead to an initial transient decrease in IOP. After GA administration (1.5–2 h), when slight conjunctival hyperemia returns, the IOP increases. It suggests a similar vasodilatation of the vascular bed of the ciliary processes causing an increase in aqueous production during the hypertensive phase. The vasodilatation can therefore be considered to be a transient α-adrenergic rebound effect after α-adrenergic stimulation, and when the pupils constrict the hypotensive phase sets in. The mechanisms which inhibit aqueous humor production seem to overlap the α-adrenergic rebound effect. It has already been mentioned that in rabbits the hypertensive response seems to be due to α-adrenergic stimulation (Langham and Krieglstein 1976). Furthermore, Unger and Hammond (1977) showed in adrenergically denervated rabbits, after pretreatment with phentolamine, an α-adrenergic blocking agent, that the hypertensive response induced with 0.1% NA disappeared. Unger and Hammond (1977) and Waitzman and Woods (1979) also showed in adrenergically denervated rabbit eyes that the hypertensive response with 0.1% NA could be blocked with indomethacin. Although these investigations were performed in rabbits and are not strictly applicable to man the following can be postulated:

2) A release of prostaglandins could be caused by α-adrenergic stimulation leading to transient disruption of the blood-aqueous barrier. This could explain the increase in aqueous humor production during the hypertensive phase with GA. Further investigations will be needed to justify this hypothesis.

Acknowledgements. We gratefully acknowledge the skillful assistance of Mrs. J. Loeb, who performed the tonometry, and Mr. A. Blijleve, who made the drawings. We thank Dispersa for providing us with Suprexon 3–0.5 (GA) during the trial.

References

Alphen GWHM van (1976) The adrenergic receptors of the intraocular muscles of the human eye. Invest Ophthalmol 15: 502–505

Holland MG, Wei CP (1973) Epinephrine dose-response characteristics of glaucomatous human eyes following chemical sympathectomy with 6-hydroxydopamine. Ann Opthalmol 5/6: 633–640

Hoyng PhFJ, Dake CL (1979) The combination of guanethidine 3% and adrenaline 0.5% in one eye drop GA in glaucoma treatment. BrJ Ophthalmol 63: 56–62

Langham ME, Krieglstein GK (1976) The biphasic intraocular pressure response of rabbits to epinephrine. Invest Ophthalmol 15: 119–127

Langham ME, Palewicz K (1977) The pupillary, the intraocular pressure and the vasomotor response to noradrenaline in rabbits. J Physiol (London) 267: 339–355

Moses RA, Becker B (1958) Clinical tonography: The sceral rigidity correction. Amer J Ophthal 45: 196–208

Unger WG, Hammond BR (1977) Noradrenaline-induced inflammation in the sympathectomized rabbit eye. IRCS Med Sci 5: 563

Waitzman MB, Woods WD (1979) Effects of prostaglandins, norepinephrine on intraocular pressure and pupil size in rabbits following cervical ganglionectomy. Invest Ophthalmol 18: 52-60

CHAPTER XI

PRODUCTION AND OUTFLOW OF THE AQUEOUS HUMOR DURING A LONG-TERM TREATMENT

PH.F.J. HOYNG & C.L. DAKE

ABSTRACT

A comparative tonographic study was performed in 10 primary open angle glaucoma patients (15 eyes) and 7 patients with suspected glaucoma (14 eyes) during a 7-months' period. The patients were treated twice daily with guanethidine 3% and adrenaline 0.5% (GA). The fall in intraocular pressure (IOP) of 44% in primary open angle glaucoma patients was mainly due to an inhibition of aqueous humour production (54%; $p < 0.005$) and to a lesser extent an increase in outflow facility. In the suspected glaucoma patients, the fall in IOP of 43% was due to an inhibition of the aqueous rate (46%; $p < 0.005$) and to an increase in outflow facility (64%; $p < 0.005$). The increase in outflow facility during treatment was significantly different between both groups of patients. It suggests degeneration of the receptors mediating outflow mechanism in the patients with open angle glaucoma. For both groups of patients it is shown that during treatment with GA there is not only a supersensitivity for adrenaline 0.5% of the mechanisms that mediate the inhibition of the aqueous rate, but also of the mechanisms that mediate outflow facility.

INTRODUCTION

During treatment of glaucoma with topical guanethidine some authors reported that the fall in intraocular pressure (IOP) was caused by an increase in outflow facility (Stepanik, 1961; Kutschera, 1961; G.D. & G. Paterson, 1972). However, other authors showed that after administration of guanethidine in eye drops, the fall in IOP was mainly due to inhibition of the aqueous humour production (Keates, 1960; Küchle, 1961; Castren, 1962; Bonomi, 1967; Merté, 1968). The fall in IOP with adrenaline is thought to be due to an initial transient inhibition of the aqueous rate (Goldmann, 1951) which is overlapped by an increase of outflow facility (Kronfeld, 1971). During administration of adrenaline for a long period, a further increase of outflow facility is reported. Becker (1958, 1961), Garner (1959) and Ballantine (1961) for instance found a gradual increase of outflow facility during long-term glaucoma treatment with adrenaline 2%. Harris (1970) and Obstbaum (1974) observed in primary open angle glaucoma patients and glaucoma suspects, respectively an increase in outflow facility after treatment with adrenaline in concentrations of 1% or more. Concentrations of less than 1% failed to increase the outflow facility and the fall in IOP was thought to be caused by inhibition of the aqueous humour production. The aim of this trial is to investigate the aqueous humour dynamics during pharmacological denervation with guanethidine and administration of adrenaline in glaucoma patients. Especially the results obtained in patients with primary open angle glaucoma were compared with those of patients suspected of having glaucoma. It is performed by means of a comparative tonographic study.

PATIENTS AND METHODS

Out of 33 patients with either primary open angle glaucoma (POAG) or suspected glaucoma, 10 POAG patients (15 eyes treated) and 7 patients with suspected glaucoma (14 eyes treated) were selected at random. During a period of 7 months the patients were treated with the combination of guanethidine 3% and adrenaline 0.5% in one eye drop (GA), twice daily at 9 a.m. and 9 p.m. (Hoyng et al., 1979). One POAG patient required additional therapy of 1 capsule diamox sustet (sustained release) and 3 x d carbachol 1½%, after treatment for a month with GA alone. In the remaining 16 patients (27 eyes) intraocular pressure was controlled with GA alone. The patients were familiar with applanation tonometry and tonography.

The criteria used for diagnosing primary open angle glaucoma and suspected glaucoma are the following. A patient was regarded POAG if the average IOP in a daycurve without medication was over 22 mm Hg, with either a visual field defect or a pathologically excavated optic disc or both, and with an open angle. A patient was regarded of having suspected glaucoma if the visual fields and the optic disc were normal, the average IOP in a daycurve without medication was over 22 mm Hg, if the IOP's were not higher than 36 mm Hg, and with an open angle. If a patient had one eye with glaucoma and the fellow eye showed only an elevated IOP, both eyes were regarded as having glaucoma.

All patients were taken off treatment one week before the trial if they had been on sympathomimetics or carbonic anydrase inhibitors, and 48 hours beforehand, if on miotics. The tonography was performed at the end of a day curve according to Grant. It was made without medication and after 1, 3 and 7 months of GA treatment. After 7 months of treatment all patients were taken off GA for 2 weeks and tonography without GA treatment was again performed. The tonography was always performed at the same time, 8 hours after GA application, and by the same investigator to eliminate undesirable fluctuations. Applanation tonometry followed by tonography was first done on the right eye and after an interval of 15 minutes on the left eye. The coefficient of outflow was calculated according to modifica-

106

tion of Mozes et al. (1958) of the Friedenwald tables. If necessary, corrections for scleral rigidity were made. The aqueous humour production was calculated with the formula $F = C (P_O - P_e)$. The applanation tonometry, taken prior to the tonography, was taken as P_O. The episcleral venous pressure was assumed to be 10 mm Hg. IOP was taken with a Goldmann applanation tonometer and the tonography was performed with the electronic Schiotz tonograph of Mueller connected with the Esterline-Angus recorder. The results were statistically evaluated by the paired t-test and by the T^2-test of Hotelling.

RESULTS

The combined results of 10 primary open angle glaucoma patients and 7 suspected glaucoma patients (29 eyes) are presented in table 1. During the 7-months' period, the fall in IOP of 44% ($p < 0.005$) is due to an increase in outflow facility of 44% ($p < 0.005$) and an inhibition of the aqueous rate of 50% ($p < 0.005$). These values were already reached after 1 month of GA treatment. After the patients had been taken off therapy for 2 weeks, IOP, outflow facility and aqueous production regained their pretreatment values.

Table 1. The mean IOP ± SEM in mm Hg, the mean coefficient of outflow (C) ± SEM in μl/min/mm Hg and the mean aqueous flow (F) ± SEM in μl/min of 10 POAG patients (15 eyes), and 7 glaucoma suspects (14 eyes).

Total

	w/o	1 Mo	3 Mo	7 Mo	w/o
Po in mm Hg ± SEM	29.9 ± 0.97	*** 16.9 ± 0.94	*** 17.4 ± 0.89	*** 17.1 ± 0.85	27.7 ± 1.48
C μl/min/mm Hg ± SEM	0.111 ± 0.010	*** 0.152 ± 0.012	*** 0.164 ± 0.014	*** 0.162 ± 0.007	0.122 ± 0.008
F μl/min ± SEM	2.08 ± 0.16	*** 0.95 ± 0.09	*** 1.07 ± 0.09	*** 1.10 ± 0.11	1.96 ± 0.10

* $p < 0.05$
** $p < 0.01$
*** $p < 0.005$

Figure 1 and table 2 present the results of the 10 primary open angle glaucoma patients alone (15 eyes). It shows that during 7 months of GA treatment, the fall in IOP of 13.9 mm Hg or 44% ($p < 0.005$) seems largely due to the inhibition of aqueous humour production of 54% ($p < 0.005$). The role of outflow facility seems to be less important in decreasing IOP, although it gradually increases from 23% ($p < 0.05$) after 1 month of GA

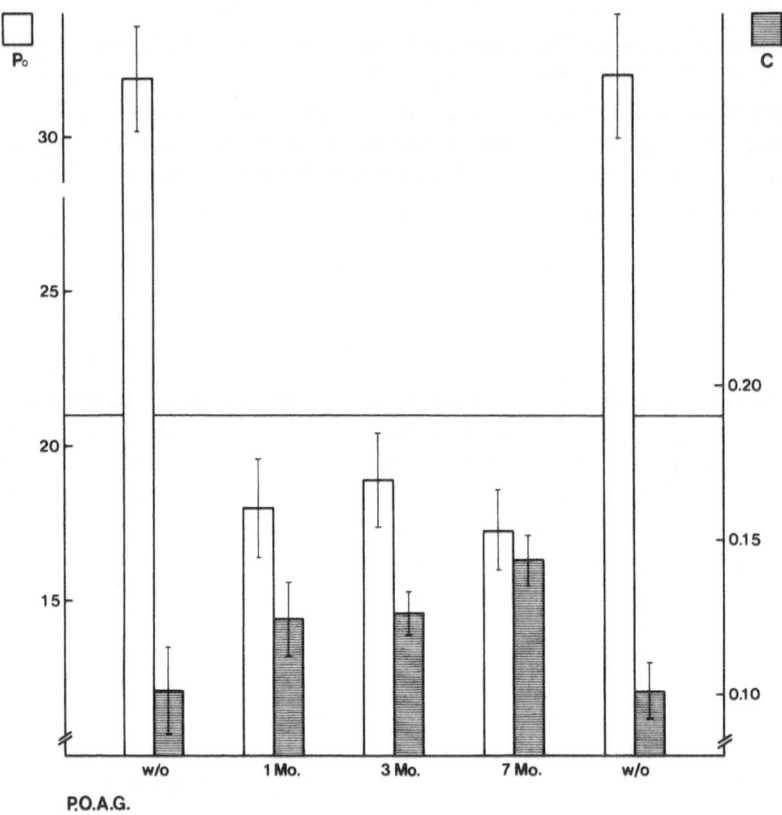

Fig. 1. The mean intraocular pressure ± SEM in mm Hg and the mean coefficient of outflow in ± SEM in μl/min/mm Hg of 10 POAG patients (15 eyes) during 7 months of GA treatment (SEM between bars).

Table 2. The mean IOP ± SEM in mm Hg, the mean coefficient of outflow (C) ± SEM in μl/min/mm Hg and the mean aqueous flow (F) ± SEM in μl/min of 10 POAG patients (15 eyes). (Significance see table 1).

10 POAG patients (n = 15)

	w/o	1 Mo	3 Mo	7 Mo	w/o
Po in mm Hg ± SEM	31.9 ± 1.67	*** 18.0 ± 1.54	*** 18.9 ± 1.48	*** 17.3 ± 1.31	32.00 ± 2.00
C μl/min/mm Hg ± SEM	0.101 ± 0.014	* 0.124 ± 0.012	* 0.126 ± 0.007	*** 0.143 ± 0.008	0.101 ± 0.009
F μl/min. ± SEM	2.07 ± 0.25	*** 0.87 ± 0.11	*** 1.03 ± 0.13	*** 0.97 ± 0.14	2.02 ± 0.07

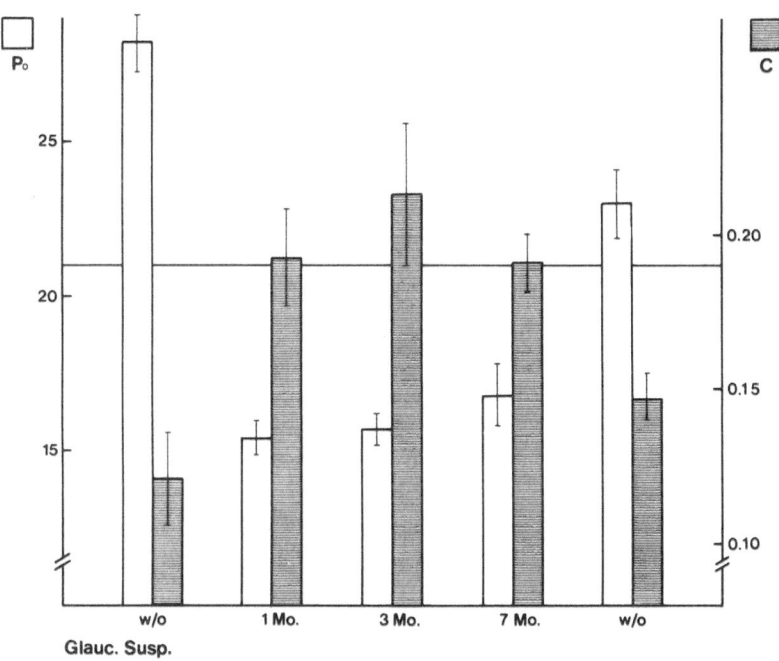

Fig. 2. The mean intraocular pressure ± SEM in mm Hg and the mean coefficient of outflow in ± SEM in μl/min/mm Hg of 7 glaucoma suspects (14 eyes) during 7 months of GA treatment (SEM between bars).

Table 3. The mean IOP ± SEM in mm Hg, the mean coefficient of outflow (C) ± SEM in μl/min/mm Hg and the mean aqueous flow (F) ± SEM μl/min of 7 suspected glaucoma patients (14 eyes). (Significance see table 1).

7 SG patients (n = 14)

	w/o	1 Mo	3 Mo	7 Mo	w/o
Po in mm Hg ± SEM	28.2 ± 0.92	*** 15.4 ± 0.49	*** 15.7 ± 0.50	*** 16.8 ± 0.99	*** 23.0 ± 1.08
C μl/min/mm Hg ± SEM	0.121 ± 0.015	*** 0.192 ± 0.015	*** 0.213 ± 0.023	*** 0.191 ± 0.009	0.147 ± 0.007
F μl/min ± SEM	2.10 ± 0.22	*** 1.06 ± 0.16	*** 1.11 ± 0.13	* 1.27 ± 0.18	1.90 ± 0.19

treatment to 43% (p < 0.005) after 7 months (increase not significant).

Pretreatment values were regained after the patients were taken off therapy for 2 weeks.

Figure 2 and table 3 show the results of 7 patients with suspected glaucoma (14 eyes). The fall in IOP of 12.2 mm Hg or 43% (p < 0.005) during the 7 months of GA treatment is due to an increase in outflow facility of 64% (p < 0.005) and an inhibition of the aqueous rate of 46% (p < 0.005). It is interesting to note that after 1 month of GA treatment the outflow facility of the suspected glaucoma group has normal values. Furthermore, after being taken off therapy for 2 weeks, there is still a fall in IOP of 5.2 mm Hg or 19% (p < 0.05).

Statistical analysis of the two groups of patients revealed no significant differences between the pretreatment values of the POAG patients and of the glaucoma suspects. Furthermore, comparing the data of each group after 1 month of treatment with those after 7 months of treatment, both groups of patients showed no trend. However, comparing the results of the POAG patients with those of the glaucoma suspects obtained after 1 month of treatment, revealed a significant difference in increasing outflow facility (p < 0.005, T^2-test of Hotelling). The data of P_O and F were not significantly different.

COMMENT

Guanethidine is thought to increase the membrane permeability of the sympathetic nerve endings resulting in a release of endogenous noradrenaline stored in the granulated vesicles of the sympathetic nerve endings. It blocks the re-uptake of noradrenaline (normally 90%), which results in a depletion of the noradrenaline stores in the sympathetic nerve endings. Supersensitivity for catecholamines develops at the receptor site. The aim of this trial was to investigate, in glaucoma patients, the mechanisms which mediate aqueous humour dynamics during pharmacological denervation with guanethidine and presumable supersensitivity for topical adrenaline 0.5%. Tonographic studies could be disturbed by different factors (Leydhecker, 1968) and the results therefore less reliable. By doing a comparative study for a long period under standardized conditions, less desirable fluctuations in episcleral venous pressure and in corneal rigidity; in pseudofacility with respect to gross facility; in uveosceral flow, and in differences between the homolateral eye and the contralateral eye, are diminished.

After 1 month of G-A treatment we found in both the patients with primary open angle glaucoma and those with suspected glaucoma, an increase in the coefficient of outflow of 23% (p < 0.05) and 59% (p < 0.005), respectively. An increase in outflow facility (significant) with adrenaline alone was found with concentrations of 1% or higher in primary open angle glaucoma patients (Harris, 1974). Furthermore no supersensitivity of

110

outflow system for adrenaline in concentrations less than 1% was reported in glaucomatous eyes after denervation with 6-hydroxyDopamine (Holland, 1973 a, b). So it is likely to conclude that, after pharmacological denervation with guanethidine, there is not only a supersensitivity for adrenaline 0.5% of the mechanisms that mediate the inhibition of the aqueous rate but also of those that mediate outflow facility in both, primary open angle glaucoma patients and those with suspected glaucoma.

In patients with suspected glaucoma, after 1 month of GA treatment, there is an increase in outflow facility compared to normal values, while in patients with established glaucoma, only a slight increase in outflow facility is observed. The difference between the two groups of patients in increasing outflow facility was significant ($p < 0.005$, T^2-test of Hotelling). It may indicate that the receptors which mediate the increase in outflow facility in POAG patients cannot react with GA in the same way as the receptors glaucoma suspects do. This could mean that established glaucoma is a pathological process in which the receptors of the outflow system have degenerated, while in glaucoma suspects the outflow is pathological, but the receptors can still function after treatment with GA, with an increase in outflow facility to normal values. This finding seems pharmacologically to enhance the study of Gwin et al. (1979), who found in the trabecular meshwork and the scleral outflow channels of beagles with POAG less intense fluorescence of adrenergic fibers compared to normal beagles, suggesting either functional or structural decrement of adrenergic fibers in beagles with POAG. In this study the adrenergic nerve fibers have been denervated with guanethidine, sothat the increase of outflow facility mainly depends upon the ability of the receptors to react on adrenaline. It is open to question whether degeneration of the receptors of the outflow system is the basic of the processes leading to established glaucoma, or that it is only a pathological condition caused by long standing elevation of IOP, as the degeneration of the axons in the nerve fiber layer of the retina. Further it is interesting to note that, in both groups of patients, the fall in IOP and the inhibition of the aqueous rate are nearly the same after 1 month of GA treatment, while the increase in outflow facility in glaucoma suspects is 3 times that of open angle glaucoma patients. It suggests that the inhibition of the aqueous production is the most important factor in lowering IOP during GA treatment. However, this study shows that the combination of guanethidine and adrenaline by its bilateral effect on both aqueous humour production and outflow, is a potential useful combination in the treatment of glaucoma patients. It further reveals a basic difference between patients with POAG and suspected glaucoma in increasing outflow facility after treatment, suggesting a pathological proces involving the receptors in the endothelial meshwork and the inner layer of Schlemms' canal in patients with POAG.

REFERENCES

Ballintine, E.J. & Garner, L.L. Improvement of the coefficient of outflow in glaucomatous eyes. *Arch. Ophthal.* 66: *314–317* (1961).

Becker, B. & Ley, A.P. Epinephrine and acetazolamide in the treatment of the chronic glaucomas. *Amer. J. Ophthal.* 45: *639–643* (1958).

Becker, B., Petitt, T.H. & Gay, A.J. Topical epinephrine therapy of open-angle glaucoma. *Arch. Ophthal.* 66: *219–225* (1961).

Becker, B. & Shin, D.H. Response to topical epinephrine. *Arch. Ophthal.* 94: *2057–2058* (1976).

Bonomi, L. & Comite, P. di. Outflow facility after guanethidine sulfate administration. *Arch. Ophthal.* 78: *337–340* (1967).

Garner, L.L. Johnstone, W.W., Ballintine, E.J. & Carroll, M.E. Effect of 2% levo-rotary epinephrine on the intraocular pressure of the glaucomatous eye. *Arch. Ophthal.* 62: *230–238* (1959).

Goldmann, H. L'origine de l'hypertension oculaire dans le glaucome primitif. *Ann. Oculist.* 184: *1086–1105* (1951).

Gwin, R.M., Gelatt, K.N. & Chiou, Ch.Y. Adrenergic and cholinergic innervation of the anterior segment of the normal and glaucomatous dog. *Invest. Ophthalmol. Vis. Sci.* 18: *674–682* (1979).

Harris, L.S., Galin, M.A. & Lerner, R. The influence of low-dose L-epinephrine on aqueous outflow facility. *Ann. Ophthal.* 2: *455–458* (1970).

Holland, M.G. & Wei, Ch.P. Epinephrine dose-response characteristics of glaucomatous human eyes following chemical sympathectomy with 6-hydroxydopamine. *Ann. Ophthal.* 5: *633–640* (1973a).

Holland, M.G. & Wei, Ch.P. Chemical sympathectomy in glaucoma therapy: An investigation of alpha and beta adrenergic supersensitivity. *Ann. Ophthal.* 5: *783–796* (1973b).

Hoyng, Ph.F.J. & Dake, C.L. The combination of guanethidine 3% and adrenaline 0.5% in one eyedrop (GA) in glaucoma treatment. *Brit. J. Ophthal.* 63: *56–62* (1979).

Keates, E.U., Narendra Krishna & Leopold, I.H. Ocular effects of guanethidine and its use in glaucoma. Symp. on Guanethidine, pp. 66–68. The University of Tennessee, College of Medicine, Memphis, Tenn. (1960).

Kronfeld, P.C. Early effects of single and repeated doses of l-epinephrine in man. *Amer. J. Ophthal.* 72: *1058* (1971).

Küchle, H.J. Zur lokalen Wirkung von Guanethidin (Ismelin) auf das gesunde und glaukomkranke Auge. *Klin. Mbl. Augenheilk.* 139: *224-234* (1961).

Kutschera, E. Klinische Erfahrungen mit Ismelin. *Klin. Mbl. Augenheilk.* 139: *234–241* (1961).

Leydhecker, W. Wert und Unwert der Tonographie. *Klin. Mbl. Augenheilk.* 153: *857–860* (1968).

Merté, H.J. & Toppel, L. Guanethidin in der Glaukomtherapie. *Graefes Arch. Ophthal.* 176: *30–42* (1968).

Obstbaum, S.A., Kolker, A.E. & Phelps, Ch.D. Low-dose epinephrine. Effect on intraocular pressure. *Arch. Ophthal.* 92: *118–120* (1974).

Paterson, G.D. & Paterson, G. Drug therapy of glaucoma. *Brit. J. Ophthal.* 56: *288–294* (1972).

Stepanik, J. Tonographische und differential tonometrische Untersuchungen über die Wirkung von Ismelin-Augentropfen (Ciba) bei Glaukoma simplex. *Graefes Arch. Ophthal.* 164: *6–9* (1961).

Maintenance Therapy of Glaucoma Patients with Guanethidine (3%) and Adrenaline (0.5%) Once Daily

Ph.F.J. Hoyng and C.L. Dake

Abstract. Over a period of 4 months, 16 of 24 patients (30 of 46 eyes) with either primary open angle glaucoma (POAG) or suspected glaucoma were treated successfully with a maintenance dose of guanethidine (3%) and adrenaline (0.5%) combined in one eyedrop (GA) once daily. In the previous month the medication was given twice daily and at the end of 4 months the decrease in intraocular pressure (IOP) was 8.9 mm Hg (33%) compared to 9.9 mm Hg (37%) with twice-daily application; three of four eyes responded just as well to single-daily application as to twice daily application of GA. Once-daily treatment with GA was not successful when the average IOP in the absence of treatment was over 32 mm Hg. The advantages of once-daily application were less conjunctival hyperemia, less dilation of the pupils, less ptosis and difficulty reading, plus the advantage that the drops needed only to be applied once a day (patient compliance). The recommended regime for GA therapy in patients with an IOP of less than 32 mm Hg is application of GA twice daily for 1 month followed by a decrease in the dosage to once a day. GA can best be applied in the evening before retiring.

Introduction

A 7-month study in which glaucoma patients were treated with the combination of guanethidine (3%) and adrenaline (0.5%) in a combined eyedrop (GA) twice daily has been reported previously (Hoyng and Dake 1979). This study revealed a fall in IOP of 10.8 mm Hg (37.5%) compared with pretreatment levels. However, side effects, such as conjunctival hyperemia, acquired hypermetropia, and ptosis were frequently seen and pupillary dilation of 2 mm or more was noted in 50% of the treated patients. Reading difficulties during the first few hours after application of GA were also reported. The main problem with the combination of guanethidine and adrenaline was not the maintenance of a lowered IOP but the side effects. The purpose of this study was to treat glaucoma suspects and patients with open angle glaucoma (POAG) with a maintenance dosage of GA once daily and to determine whether once-daily application of GA was therapeutically effective and whether it cut down the incidence of side effects.

The results in POAG patients were compared with those obtained from the glaucoma suspects and also compared with the results of the 7-month study of twice-daily application. In order to get an accurate impression of the effects of once-daily GA on IOP, supplemental treatment was avoided as much as possible.

Materials and Methods

Twelve POAG patients and 12 glaucoma suspects were selected at random from a previously described study on glaucoma patients (Hoyng and Dake 1979). These patients had been treated with twice-daily GA for 7 months. After a period of 14 days without medication, a day curve was obtained and the patients resumed treatment with twice-daily GA for 1 month. Thereafter they were shifted to once-daily GA (at 5 p.m.) and a second day curve was obtained 1 week later. The first measurement at zero time (9 a.m.) showed the IOP 16 h after the last application of GA. Since no GA was administered during the day curve, the course of IOP 16–24 h after the last application of GA was established. At the beginning of the study, one POAG patient received pilocarpine (2%) four times a day and sustained-release Diamox once daily while one glaucoma suspect received pilocarpine (2%) twice daily as supplemental treatment. No additional supplemental treatment was given during the study and patients whose IOP could not be controlled on once-daily GA were eliminated from the trial. After approximately 4 months (4.2 ± 1.98 SD) on this treatment, the IOP day curve was repeated. The results of this study then compared with the results in the same patients after 7 months on twice-daily GA.

After the treatment with twice-daily GA for 7 months, medication had been withdrawn for 2 weeks. Nevertheless, in many patients the IOP was still noticeably affected by GA. Hence the initial day curves (without medication) taken before the study with twice-daily GA were used. The average IOP and decrease in IOP in mm Hg and as a percentage were calculated from the measurements at 0, 3, 6, and 8 h. Visual acuity, refraction, and IOP were checked monthly during a brief visit to the outpatient clinic and the patients were examined for (and questioned about) the presence of side effects.

IOP was considered to be well-controlled if all IOP's were lower than 22 mm Hg, and controlled if, in a day curve, all IOP's but one were lower than 22 mm Hg and not higher than 25 mm Hg. IOP was not controlled if, in a day curve, more than one IOP was higher than 21 mm Hg or one IOP was higher than 25 mm Hg. The results were statistically evaluated with the aid of paired t-test.

Results

In 5 of the 12 POAG patients the IOP was not considered to be controlled after 1 week on once-daily GA and treatment was discontinued. In a sixth POAG patient the treatment with GA was discontinued in one eye due to high pressures and replaced by pilocarpine (2%) four times a day. The average decrease in IOP in the 12 POAG patients was 8.8 mm Hg (29%) ($P < 0.005$) after 1 week on once-daily GA compared to 11.6 mm Hg (38%) after treatment with twice-daily GA (Table 1).

In 2 of the 12 glaucoma suspects, treatment with once-daily GA was stopped after 1 week because IOP became uncontrolled. In a third glaucoma suspect

Table 1. Mean IOP ± SEM (mm Hg) with and without guanethidine and adrenaline (GA) in 12 primary open angle glaucoma (POAG) patients and 12 glaucoma suspects, as well as in 16 patients whose IOP was controlled, compared to nine patients whose IOP was not controlled

	Without medication	After 7 months GA (2 × day)			After 1 week GA (1 × day)			After 4 months GA (1 × day)		
	Mean IOP ± SEM	Mean IOP ± SEM	ΔP (mm Hg)	ΔP (%)	Mean IOP ± SEM	ΔP (mm Hg)	ΔP (%)	Mean IOP ± SEM	ΔP (mm Hg)	ΔP (%)
12 POAG patients (N = 22)	30.4 ± 0.90	18.7[a] ± 0.44	11.6	38	21.6[a] ± 0.62	8.8	29	—	—	—
12 glaucoma suspects (N = 24)	26.5 ± 0.45	17.4[a] ± 0.34	9	34	17.9[a] ± 0.53	8.6	32	18.3[a] ± 0.42	8.2	31
Six POAG patients + three glaucoma suspects (N = 16)	31.3 ± 1.19	19.6[a] ± 0.48	11.7	37.5	24.9[a] ± 0.61	6.4	21	—	—	—
Nine glaucoma suspects + seven POAG patients (N = 30)	27.0 ± 0.38	17.1[a] ± 0.29	9.9	37	16.7[a] ± 0.33	10.3	38	18.1[a] ± 0.32	8.9	33

[a] $P < 0.005$

115

Table 2. Relation of the mean IOP without medication to the mean IOP during treatment with once-daily guanethidine + adrenaline (GA)

Mean IOP (mm Hg) without medication	< 24 mm Hg	24–28 mm Hg	28–32 mm Hg	> 32 mm Hg
Well controlled	2	13	7	–
Controlled	–	2	5	1
Not controlled	3	5	2	6

(receiving supplemental treatment) the ocular pressure became uncontrolled after 4 months on once-daily GA. After 1 week on once-daily GA, the average IOP of the 12 glaucoma suspects was 17.9 mm Hg and the decrease in ocular pressure was 8.6 mm Hg (32%) ($P < 0.005$). After 4 month treatment with once-daily GA, the remaining ten glaucoma suspects had an average IOP of 18.3 mm Hg and a decrease in ocular pressure of 8.2 mm Hg (31%) ($P < 0.005$) compared to a decrease of 9 mm Hg (34%) after treatment with GA twice daily (Table 1).

Figure 1 and Table 1 show the results in nine glaucoma suspects and seven POAG patients (30 eyes) in whom the treatment was successful. After 4 months with once daily GA, the average IOP was 18.1 mm Hg and the average decrease in ocular pressure was 8.9 mm Hg (33%) ($P < 0.005$). There was hardly any difference between these results and those of twice-daily GA.

Figure 2 and Table 1 show the results in six POAG patients (ten eyes) and three glaucoma suspects (six eyes) whose IOP was not controlled on once-daily GA. The day curves without medication show that these were patients with initially higher IOP. After 1 week of treatment there was still a decrease in IOP of 6.4 mm Hg (21%) ($P < 0.005$).

Table 2 shows the average IOP in the absence of treatment for each patient in relation to the degree of control on once-daily GA. In Table 3 the degree of control on once-daily GA for each patient is compared with the control achieved after 7 months on GA twice daily. Patients who were almost controlled on twice-daily GA (i.e., one IOP reading greater than 21 mm Hg but not 25 mm Hg) were the ones who developed higher IOP on once-daily GA. Patients who were well-controlled on twice-daily GA also showed well-regulated IOP with once-daily application.

Table 4 shows the side effects during treatment with GA twice-daily and with GA once-daily for ten glaucoma suspects and seven POAG patients. The visual acuity and refraction remained unchanged during the entire 4-month period. The decrease in side effects during once-daily application of GA was striking.

Discussion

Guanethidine is thought to increase the membrane permeability of the sympathetic nerve endings, leading to release of the noradrenaline (NA) stored in the granulated vesicles. It also blocks the reuptake of NA, resulting in depletion

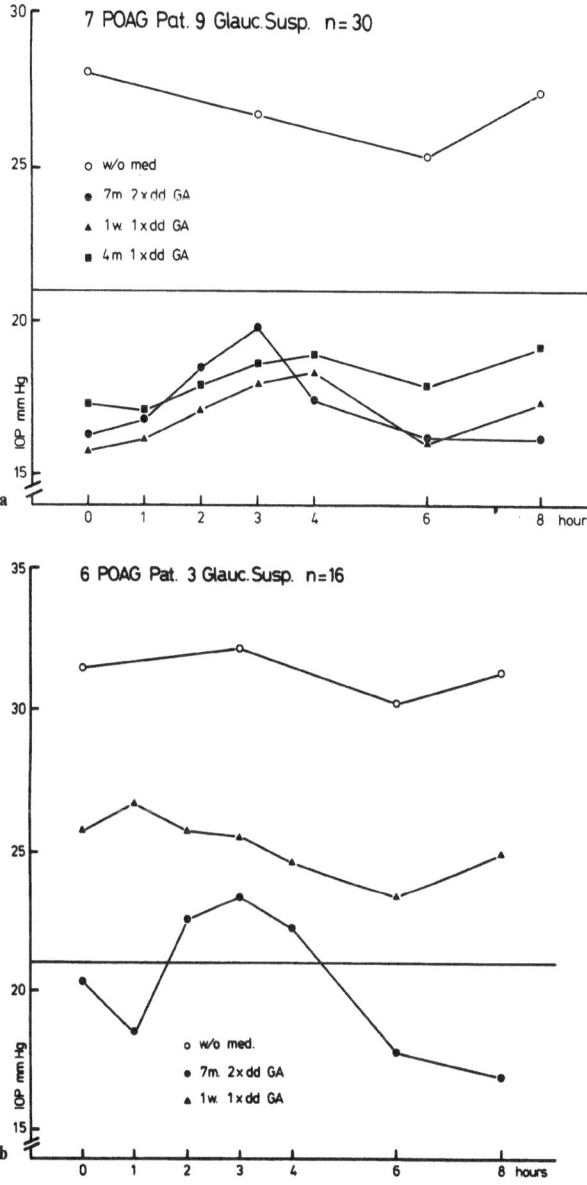

Fig. 1a and b. Mean IOP day-curve with and without therapy, with once-daily guanethidine+ adrenaline (GA) after 1 week or 4 months (measurements 16-24 h after the last application of GA), and with twice-daily GA after 7 months (measurements 0-8 h after the last application of GA) in 16 patients whose IOP was controlled (a) and in nine patients whose IOP was not controlled (b) on once-daily GA.

117

Table 3. Comparison of the results with once-daily and twice-daily guanethidine + adrenaline (GA) in 24 glaucoma patients (46 eyes)

	After 7 months GA (2 × day)		After 4 months GA (1 × day)	
	Number of eyes	Percent	Number of eyes	Percent
Well controlled	25	54	22	48
Controlled	16	35	8	17
Not controlled	5	11	16	35

Table 4. Comparison of the side effects in 17 patients during treatment with guanethidine + adrenaline (GA) once and twice daily

	After 7 months of GA (2 × day)	After 4 months of GA (1 × day)
Drops unpleasant	1	—
Burning sensations	1	—
Foreign body sensations	1	—
Reading problems	4	1
Ptosis (slight or transient)	2	—
Hyperemia		
Slight	8	4
Medium	1	—
Kerato epitheliopathy	—	—

of the NA stores in the sympathetic nerve endings. Hypersensitivity to catechol-amines, therefore, develops in the sympathetically denervated receptor (Mitchell and Oates 1970).

After pharmacological denervation, the hypersensitivity of the adrenergic receptor is manifested after administration of adrenaline by a more pronounced decrease in ocular pressure, ascribable mainly to the hypersensitivity of the mechanisms affecting in the inhibition of the production of aqueous humor (Holland 1973a, b). It has been demonstrated (Hoyng and Dake, work in progress) that in glaucoma patients treated with GA twice-daily the mechanisms mediating outflow facility were also hypersensitive to adrenaline. Hence, the combination of guanethidine and adrenaline has a double effect on the ocular pressure due to a marked inhibition of the production of aqueous humor together with an increase in outflow facility. When the combined GA eyedrop is applied once a day, the question arise as to whether a drop of guanethidine (3%) once every 24 h can maintain a denervated state and create sufficient hypersensi-tivity to adrenergic agents, and whether application of 0.5% adrenaline only once every 24 h can maintain a therapeutic decrease in IOP. In relation to these questions, the levels of IOP 16–24 h after application of GA seemed to be the most important. In view of the results with twice-daily application of GA, a preliminary period of 1 month on twice-daily GA seems adequate as an introduction to once-daily application. The results of the present study show that 48% of the eyes were well controlled and 65% were controlled after 4 months on once-daily GA compared to 54% and 89%, respectively, after twice-daily application of GA. In three of every four eyes treated with GA twice daily, the medication needed only to be applied once a day. The course of the IOP day curve is much more constant on once-daily GA due to the elimination of one hypertensive response. It can be seen from Table 2 that patients with an average IOP higher than 32 mm Hg should not be considered for once-daily treatment, but treatment with GA once daily is adequate whenever the average IOP, in the absence of treatment, is lower than 32 mm Hg.

Glaucoma suspects do not seem to respond any better to once-daily application of GA than patients with POAG, especially in view of the fact that the patients with POAG had higher IOP in this study. It would seem, therefore, that the level of IOP in the absence of treatment is the best criterion for determining whether or not maintenance therapy with once-daily GA will be successful. Table 4 shows that side effects decreased significantly. The fact that the medication only needed be applied once a day, combined with less conjunctival hyperemia, fewer reading difficulties, and an absence of ptosis contributed to patient compliance. On the basis of this study it is concluded that the most suitable technique for using GA is to begin with twice-daily application for 1 month followed by maintenance therapy with GA once a day. If the medication is applied just before retiring, then the transitory ptosis and dilation of the pupils occur while the patient is asleep and are, therefore, not troublesome. A patient with an initial IOP lower than 32 mm Hg can be kept under acceptable control with once-daily application when the medication is used in this way.

Acknowledgement. We gratefully acknowledge the skillful assistance of Mrs. J. Loeb, who performed the tonometry, and Mr. A. Blijleve, who made the drawings. We thank Dispersa for providing us with Suprexon 3–0.5 (GA) during the trial.

References

Holland MG, Wei CP (1973a) Epinephrine dose-response characteristics of glaucomatous human eyes following chemical sympathectomy with 6-hydroxydopamine. Ann Ophthalmol 5/6:633–640

Holland MG, Wei, CP (1973b) Chemical sympathectomy in glaucoma. Therapy: An investigation of alpha- and beta-adrenergic supersensitivity. Ann Ophthalmol 5/7:783–796

Hoyng PFJ, Dake CL (1979) The combination of guanethidine (3%) and adrenaline (0.5%) in 1 eyedrop (GA) in glaucoma treatment. Br J Ophthalmol 63:56–62

Mitchell JR, Oates, JA (1970) Guanethidine and related agents. Mechanism of the selective blockade of adrenergic neurons and its antagonism by drugs. J Pharmacol Exp Ther 172:100–107

CHAPTER XIII

THE COMBINATION OF GUANETHIDINE 1% AND EPINEPHRINE 0.2% IN ONE EYE DROP (GA-WEAK) IN THE TREATMENT OF GLAUCOMA

PH.F.J. HOYNG & C.L. DAKE

ABSTRACT

Thirty-one patients (58 eyes) with either primary open angle glaucoma (19 patients with 34 eyes) or suspected glaucoma (12 patients with 24 eyes) were treated for a period of 7 months with only guanethidine 1% and epinephrine 0.2% in one eyedrop (GA-weak) twice daily. The intraocular pressure (IOP) was controlled in 64% of all eyes with an average pressure decrease of 8.4 mm Hg or 31% (p < 0.005). Tonography revealed that the decrease in IOP was due both to inhibition of aqueous humour production (26%, p < 0.005) and to an increase in outflow facility (32%, p < 0.005), showing supersensitivity to inflow and outflow for epinephrine 0.2%. 8 patients were eliminated from the study due to tolerance for the drug.

The side-effects were mild and did not lead to cessation of treatment. GA-weak was found to be an effective agent in the management of glaucoma. The treatment was well tolerated by the patients.

INTRODUCTION

The combination of guanethidine and epinephrine in one eyedrop has been available for the treatment of glaucoma since 1976. Jones (Jones et al., 1977) reported that guanethidine 5% and epinephrine 1% in one eyedrop produced a 10% greater decrease in intraocular pressure (IOP) than either of the drugs separately applicated. The combination of guanethidine 3% and adrenaline 0.5% in one eyedrop did not produce a greater decrease in IOP but did yield fewer side-effects. We studied the effects of guanethidine 3% and epinephrine 0.5% in one eyedrop (GA-medium) in glaucoma patients over a long period and observed a decrease in IOP of 10.8 mm Hg or 37.5% (Hoyng & Dake, 1979). This decrease was caused both by an inhibition of aqueous humour production (50%) and by an increase in outflow facility (44%) (Hoyng, 1980).

Nagasubramanian (Nagasubramanian et al., 1976) treated glaucoma patients with guanethidine 1% and epinephrine 0.005-0.5% in separate eyedrops as supplemental therapy. They reported an extra decrease in IOP of 9 mm Hg in 95% of their patients without any side-effects.

Whenever patients are treated with a lower concentration of a drug, the incidence of undesirable side-effects will normally decrease. The question, however, is whether or not the intended effect is maintained and whether the development of tolerance may not be facilitated.

The purpose of this study was to treat glaucoma patients exclusively with guanethidine 1% and epinephrine 0.2% (GA-weak) twice daily for a long period. No additional therapy was permitted, so that the effect of GA-weak on IOP and aqueous humour dynamics, together with the side-effects produced by this agent, could be clearly delineated and the suitability of this eyedrop could be evaluated.

PATIENTS AND METHODS

Thirty-one patients (22 men and 9 women) with either primary open angle glaucoma (POAG) (19 patients, 34 eyes) or suspected glaucoma (12 patients, 24 eyes) were admitted to the study. The average age was 62 years (range 42-79 years) and the treatment lasted for an average of 7 months (range 1-12 months). The patients were ambulatory and had been referred to the glaucoma department for evaluation and treatment of their disease by other ophthalmologists. This implies that they were accustomed to tonometry. The criteria used for the diagnosis of POAG or suspected glaucoma have been described in detail elsewhere (Hoyng & Dake, 1979). Before the patients were admitted to the study the ophthalmological and general case histories were recorded and an ophthalmological examination was carried out. Patients who were receiving oral treatment with β-blockers, α-methyldopa, reserpine, Ismelin or tricyclic anti-depressants were excluded. The ophthalmological examination included visual acuity and refraction, biomicroscopy with the Haag-Streit Slit-lamp, gonioscopy with Goldmann's three-mirror contactglass and binocular examination of the papilla and blood vessels. Static and kinetic perimetry with the aid of the Tübingen and Goldmann perimeters, respectively, were performed before and after the study for evaluation of the visual field.

In all patients the previous treatment was discontinued at least 48 hours prior to the study if they were receiving miotic agents and one week before if they were receiving sympathomimetic agents or carbonic anhydrase inhibitors. Patients who had already been treated with guanethidine 3% and epinephrine 0.5% in one eyedrop were treated with pilocarpine 2% 4x daily during a washout period of at least one month before a day-curve in the absence of therapy was recorded. The previous therapy received by all patients is summarized in table 1. After a day-curve in the absence of therapy was recorded for all patients, at least 4 measurements being made at 9.00 a.m. and 12.00 noon (0-3 hours) and at 3.00 p.m. and 5.00 p.m. (6-8 hours), they were started on the combination of guanethidine 1% and

122

Table 1. Previous therapy of 31 patients (58 eyes).

	Number of eyes
Pilocarpine 2% 4xd	18
Guanethidine 3%-Epinephrine 0.5% 1xd	21
Epinephrine borate 1% 2xd	4
Ocusert P-40	2
Acetazolamide sustained release 1xd	2
Acetazolamide 0.250	3
None	16

epinephrine 0.2% in one eyedrop (suprexon 1-0,2) twice daily at 9.00 a.m. and 9.00 p.m. provided they had during the day-curve without medication at least one IOP reading over 25 mm Hg or a mean IOP over 22 mm Hg. The day-curves were repeated after 1, 4 and 7 months of treatment. GA-weak was always applied immediately after the first measurement, so that the first measurement at zero-time indicated the IOP 12 hours after the last application. No supplemental therapy was permitted in this study, so that if in a patient the IOP was not regulated he was eleminated. Every 6 weeks throughout the study, the patients reported to the out-patient clinic for control of the visual acuity, refraction and IOP and to be questioned about possible side-effects. During the IOP day-curve made after one month of treatment the pupil size was measured with a millimeter ruler under standardized illumination to the nearest 0.5 mm.

The patients were considered to be 'well controlled' if all IOP values were lower than 22 mm Hg, 'controlled' if all but one of the IOP values in the day-curve were lower than 22 mm Hg and the exception was not higher than 25 mm Hg, and 'not controlled' if in a day-curve more than one of the IOP values were higher than 21 mm Hg or one higher than 25 mm Hg. The IOP was measured with a Goldmann applanation tonometer mounted on a Haag-Streit Slit-lamp.

Out of the group of 31 patients, 14 (6 glaucoma suspects with 12 eyes and 8 POAG patients with 15 eyes) were selected at random and also subjected to tonography according to Grant. This was carried out with a Mueller electronic-Schiøtz tonograph just before and at the end of the study, after a day-curve had been recorded. The coefficient of outflow was calculated according to the modification of Moses of the Friedenwald tables. If necessary, corrections for scleral rigidity were made. The episcleral venous pressure was assumed to be 10 mm Hg. The results were evaluated statistically by means of paired t-test.

RESULTS

In 19 patients (11 POAG patients and 8 glaucoma suspects) the IOP remained controlled during the study; of these one POAG patient died suddenly after 5 months of treatment. The average day-curves of these patients are shown

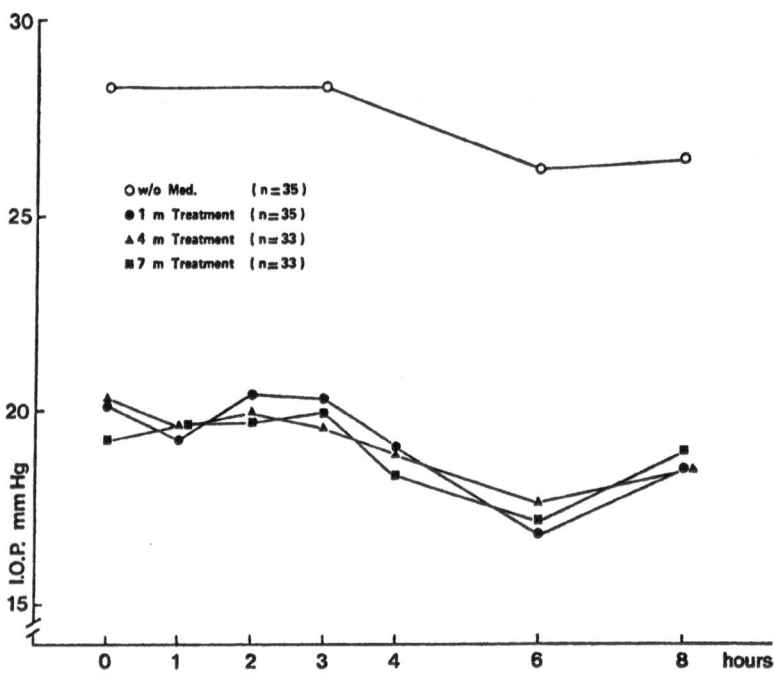

Fig. 1. Mean IOP day-curves with and without treatment of 19 glaucoma patients (35 eyes) who were successfully treated with GA-weak twice daily.

Table 2. The results of successful treatment of 19 glaucoma patients (35 eyes), in mm Hg ± standard error of the mean (SEM).

Hours	0	1	2	3	4	6	8
Mean IOP in mm Hg without medication (n=35)	28.3 0.83			28.3 0.64		26.2 0.66	26.4 1.02
Mean IOP in mm Hg after 1 month of treatment (n=35)	20.1 0.65	19.3 0.50	20.4 0.54	20.3 0.53	19.0 0.62	16.9 0.47	18.5 0.47
Mean IOP in mm Hg after 4 months of treatment (n=33)	20.2 0.49	19.5 0.48	19.9 0.41	19.5 0.39	18.9 0.48	17.6 0.44	18.5 0.58
Mean IOP in mm Hg after 7 months of treatment (n=33)	19.2 0.54	19.5 0.49	19.8 0.36	19.8 0.45	18.3 0.48	17.1 0.43	18.9 0.52

124

in figure 1 and table 2. The average decrease in IOP was 8.4 mm Hg or 31% (p < 0.005) and was already achieved after one month of treatment.

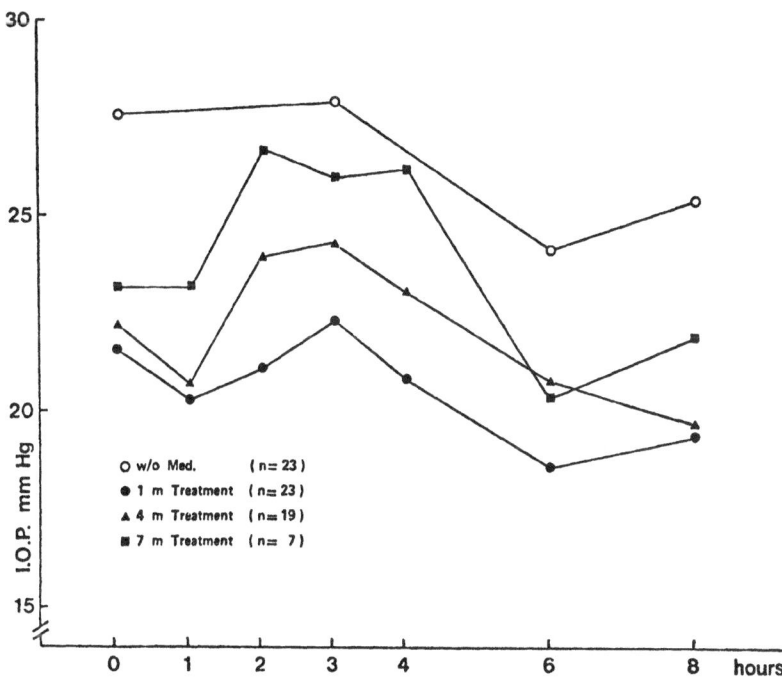

Fig. 2. Mean IOP day-curves with and without treatment of 12 glaucoma patients (23 eyes) who were not regulated during the trial.

Table 3. The results of treating 12 glaucoma patients (23 eyes) who were not regulated, in mm Hg ± SEM.

Hours	0	1	2	3	4	6	8
Mean IOP in mm Hg without medication (n=23)	27.6 0.90			27.9 0.87		24.2 0.97	25.4 0.67
Mean IOP in mm Hg after 1 month of treatment (n=23)	21.6 0.89	20.3 1.03	21.1 0.63	22.3 0.75	20.9 0.60	18.6 0.69	19.4 0.72
Mean IOP in mm Hg after 4 months of treatment (n=19)	22.1 0.76	20.6 0.61	23.9 0.99	24.2 1.20	23.0 0.80	20.7 0.80	19.6 0.69
Mean IOP in mm Hg after 7 months of treatment (n=7)	23.1 1.14	23.1 0.60	26.6 0.95	25.9 2.27	26.1 1.77	20.4 0.37	21.9 0.96

During the first 2 months of treatment, 2 POAG patients and 2 glaucoma suspects were eliminated from the study due to insufficient decrease in IOP. Subsequently in the next period of treatment an additional 8 patients (6 POAG patients and 2 glaucoma suspects) left the study due to drug tolerance.

Figure 2 and table 3 show the results in the 12 patients (8 POAG patients and 4 glaucoma suspects) who were not controlled. The average decrease in IOP in this group was 5.7 mm Hg or 21% ($p < 0.005$) after one month of treatment, 4.7 mm Hg or 17.9% ($p < 0.005$) after 4 months and 3.5 mm Hg or 13.3% ($p < 0.005$) after 7 months. The course of the IOP day-curves and the number of eyes treated reveals the development of tolerance for GA-weak.

Table 4 shows the results of tonography in 14 patients (8 POAG patients and 6 glaucoma suspects) before and after treatment with GA-weak. It appears that the decrease in IOP (27%, $p < 0.005$) was due to a 32% increase in outflow facility ($p < 0.005$) and a 26% inhibition of aqueous humour production ($p < 0.005$). In 4 patients of this group, all with POAG, the ocular pressure was no longer under control; this failure can be ascribed to tolerance of inflow and outflow mechanisms for GA-weak. During the first four months of treatment these patients responded well.

Table 4. The results of tonography in 6 patients suspected of having glaucoma and 8 patients with POAG. Po in mm Hg $\pm$ SEM, the mean coefficient of outflow (C) in μl/min/mm Hg $\pm$ SEM, and flow (F) in μl/min $\pm$ SEM. Significance is indicated in the text.

	Without medication			After treatment		
	P_O	C	F	P_O	C	F
				***	***	***
8 POAG + 6 glaucoma	26.7	0.12	2.00	19.6	0.16	1.49
suspects (27 eyes)	0.77	0.008	0.13	0.56	0.009	0.09
				***	**	**
4 POAG + 6 glaucoma suspects	27.8	0.13	2.21	19.1	0.18	1.57
(controlled, 19 eyes)	0.89	0.010	0.16	0.64	0.010	0.12
4 POAG	23.9	0.11	1.52	20.6	0.13	1.31
(uncontrolled, 8 eyes)	0.96	0.008	0.10	1.10	0.016	0.14

* indicates $p < 0.05$

** indicates $p < 0.01$

*** indicates $p < 0.005$

The degree to which the ocular pressure was controlled is summarized for all patients in table 5. In 40% of the treated eyes all IOP values were lower than 22 mm Hg while in an additional 24% all IOP values but one were lower than 22 mm Hg and the one exception was not higher than 25 mm Hg.

Table 5. Number of eyes and percentage regulated by GA-weak.

	Number of eyes	%
Well controlled	23	40
Controlled	14	24
Not controlled	21	36

Table 6 demonstrated that the success or failure of treatment with GA-weak does not seem to depend on the initial height of the IOP (mean of the day-curve without medication).

Table 6. Relation of the IOP in the absence of therapy to the IOP during treatment of the individual eyes.

Mean IOP without medication	<24 mm Hg	24-28 mm Hg	28-32 mm Hg	$\geqslant 32$ mm Hg
Well controlled	5	10	3	5
Controlled	2	8	3	1
Not controlled	3	12	5	1

Side-effects in 31 patients during treatment with GA-weak by itself:

None of the patients found the treatment unpleasant or complained of burning, stabbing pains, brow-ache, epiphora or foreignbody sensations. A very mild conjunctival hyperaemia was noted by the author in 9 patients, 2 of whom had also noticed it themselves. Mild or transient ptosis (1-2 mm) was seen in 2 patients and moderate ptosis (2-3 mm) in one. After instillation of GA-weak 26% of the eyes showed a slight dilatation of the pupil (2-3 mm) only. Three patients complained of reading difficulties during the first few hours after application of GA-weak. No keratoepitheliopathy was noted. There were also no significant changes in visual acuity, refraction or the visual fields.

DISCUSSION

Guanethidine is thought to increase the membrane permeability of the sympathetic nerve endings resulting in a release of endogenous norepinephrine stored in the granulated vesicles. It blocks the re-uptake of norepinephrine (normally 90%) leading to depletion of the norepinephrine stores in the sympathetic nerve endings (Mitchell & Oates, 1970). As result the receptors are rendered supersensitive for direct acting sympathomimetic agents. In a pharmacological denervated eye this supersensitivity is manifested by, among other things, a more pronounced decrease in ocular pressure after application of an agent such as epinephrine. The more pronounced decrease in IOP is mainly due to supersensitivity of the mechanisms that mediate the inhibition of the aqueous humour formation and not to supersensitivity of the mechanisms that mediate outflow facility (Holland & Wei, 1973).

An increase in outflow facility with epinephrine alone is reported with concentrations of 1% or higher in patients with POAG (Harris, Galin & Lerner, 1970) and in patients suspected of having glaucoma (Obstbaum, Kolker & Phelps, 1974). From the present study it is apparent that during denervation with topical guanethidine 1% both the mechanisms that mediate the inhibition of the aqueous humour formation as well as the mechanisms that mediate the increase in outflow facility, are supersensitive to epinephrine in concentrations of 0.2%. By its bilateral effect on aqueous humour dynamics GA-weak is a potent drug in the management of glaucoma.

The problems during the treatment of glaucoma patients with guanethidine and epinephrine are not so much an insufficient decrease in IOP but rather undesirable side-effects such as conjunctival hyperaemia, ptosis and keratoepitheliopathy. The combination of both agents in one eyedrop, together with a reduction in the concentration of each agent, is designed to reduce these side-effects. In experiments on the nictating membrane of cats it was shown that a longterm low dose of reserpine (0.1 mg/Kg) injected daily produced the same amount of supersensitivity (Fleming & Trendelenburg, 1961) and the same amount of depletion of norepinephrine (Trendelenburg & Weiner, 1962) as one single large dose (3 mg/Kg). So it seemed justified to reduce the concentration of a denervating agent. In view of this the concentration of guanethidine was lowered to 1%.

Smith (1976) pointed to the fact that in glaucoma treatment 'the mean IOP is of little importance since it may be weighted with numerous normal readings'. Therefore a 'normal' mean IOP in a day-curve during treatment is not a parameter for regulating an elevated IOP. For this reason, in our model (described in materials and methods) peaks were not eliminated.

In this study 64% of the eyes was succesfully treated with GA-weak showing an average decrease in IOP of 8.4 mm Hg or 31%. Although the decrease in IOP produced by GA-weak is somewhat smaller than that with GA-medium, the side-effects are also fewer.

Furthermore, with GA-medium twice daily, the IOP showed a biphasic course (Hoyng & Dake, 1979). Approximately 3 hours after application of GA-medium, the IOP peaked at 3.5 mm Hg (p < 0.005) above the hypotensive phase. This 3-hour peak was caused by a 36% increase in aqueous humour production and not by fluctuations in the coefficient of outflow (Hoyng, in preparation). During treatment with GA-weak, a similar biphasic pattern appears only in the patients who are not controlled (see fig. 2, the day-curves after 4 and 7 months). Due to the absence of such a biphasic pattern in the patients who are treated successfully, the course of the IOP is much more constant.

Glaucoma suspects seem to respond better to GA-weak than patients with POAG. The success or failure of treatment with GA-weak does not seem to be determined by the height of the IOP at the beginning of treatment (see table VI). The patients were pleased that the agent had to be applied only twice daily and the few side-effects were never a reason to stop treatment.

During the treatment with GA-medium twice daily, tolerance developed in only 1 of 33 patients (Hoyng & Dake, 1979). (We prefer to use the word tolerance instead of tachyphylaxis or adaptation). These findings can be contrasted with the results of the present study, in which 8 of the 31 patients developed tolerance. It leads to the conclusion that a reduction in the concentration of guanethidine and epinephrine may lead to a certain degree of tolerance.

In view of the results of treating glaucoma with timolol, it is interesting to compare GA-weak and timolol 0.5%. Especially the control of glaucoma was tested with the above described model. In a comparative study on 18 glaucoma patients there was no significant difference between both drugs in decreasing IOP, in regulating glaucoma and in the development of drug tolerance. The side-effects however were less with timolol (Hoyng, 1980).

In summary, glaucoma can be well regulated with GA-weak twice daily although one should be aware of the fact that tolerance may develop in a proportion of the patients (26% in the present study).

ACKNOWLEDGEMENTS

We gratefully acknowledge the skillful assistance of Mrs. J. Loeb, who performed the tonometry, and Mr. A. Blijleve, who made the drawings.

We thank ZYMA and BAESCHLIN for providing us with suprexon 1-0.2 (GA-weak) during the trial.

REFERENCES

Fleming, W.W. & Trendelenburg, U. Development of supersensitivity to norepinephrine after pretreatment with reserpine. *J. Pharm. Exp. Ther.* 133: *41–51* (1961).

Harris, L.S., Galin, M.A. & Lerner, R. The influence of low-dose 1-epinephrine on intraocular pressure. *Ann. Ophthal.* 2: *253–257* (1970).

Holland, M.G. & Wei, Ch.P. Epinephrine dose-response characteristics of glaucomatous human eye following chemical sympathectomy with 6-hydroxydopamine. *Ann. Ophthal.* 5: *633–640* (1973).

Hoyng, Ph.F.J. Adrenergic therapy in glaucoma, especially the combination of guanethidine and adrenaline in one eyedrop. *Docum. Ophthal. Proc. Ser.* 22: *303–312* (1980).

Hoyng, Ph.F.J. & Dake, C.L. The combination of guanethidine 3% and adrenaline 0.5% in one eyedrop (GA) in glaucoma treatment. *Brit. J. Ophthal.* 63: *56–62* (1979).

Jones, D.E.P., Norton, D.A. & Davies, D.J.G. Low dosage combined adrenaline-guanethidine formulations in the management of chronic simple glaucoma. *Trans. Ophthal. Soc. U.K.* 97: *192–196* (1977).

Mitchell, J.R. & Oates, J.A. Guanethidine and related agents. I: Mechanisms of selective blockade of adrenergic neurons and its antagonism by drugs. *J. Pharm. Exp. Ther.* 172: *100–107* (1970).

Nagasubramanian, S., Tripathi, R.C., Poinoosawny, D. & Gloster, J. Low concentration guanethidine and adrenaline therapy in glaucoma. *Trans. Ophthal. Soc. U.K.* 96: *179–183* (1976).

Obstbaum, S.A., Kolker, A.E. & Phelps, Ch.D. Low dose epinephrine. Effect on intraocular pressure. *Arch. Ophthal.* 92: *118–120* (1974).

Smith, R. Medical versus surgical therapy in glaucoma patients. *Docum. Ophthal. Proc. Ser.* 12: *123–131* (1976).

Trendelenburg, U. & Weiner, N. Sensitivity of the nictating membrane after various procedures and agents. *J. Pharm. Exp. Ther.* 136: *151–161* (1962).

CHAPTER XIV

ADRENERGIC THERAPY IN GLAUCOMA, ESPECIALLY THE COMBINATION OF GUANETHIDINE AND ADRENALINE IN ONE EYEDROP

ABSTRACT

Adrenaline (epinephrine), dipivalyl epinephrine and guanethidine eyedrops will be discussed. Mechanisms, short and long-term effects, side effects will be considered.

Adrenaline and guanethidine combined in one eye drop is a promising drug; the mechanism of action is based on supersensitivity to adrenaline caused by guanethidine. The average reduction of intraocular pressure is approximately 35%. Side effects will be compared with those of other drugs.

Interesting aspects are the differences between primary open angle glaucoma and suspects (ocular hypertensives) and the biphasic response to this drug combination. Some speculations for future developments are given.

The topical treatment of glaucoma can be divided into treatment with miotics and treatment with non-miotics.

The side-effects and complications with miotic therapy are as follows:

– miosis, dark vision, blurred vision (cataract).

– ciliary spasm, accomodation, myopia, browache.

– red eyes.

– sphincter rigidity, posterior synechiae, iris cysts.

– ablatio.

– angle closure.

However, miotics are indispensable in the presence of a narrow angle or narrow angle component, if a periferal iridectomy has not been performed. Treatment with non-miotics does not result in side-effects such as miosis, dark illumination, myopia or blurred vision. The frequency of application is twice daily at most, which implies that the patient does not have to use eyedrops during office hours.

Many of the agents in this group dilate the pupils. Therefore the categorization 'non-miotic' implies that the angle must be open. The ophthalmologist may be reminded of this by dilation of the pupil. If this sign is lacking, such as during treatment with β-blockers, and if no gonioscopy has been performed, then a narrow angle component may remain undetected and hence untreated. Consequently, gonioscopy must be performed in every glaucoma patient treated with non-miotic drugs.

The non-miotics can be divided into:

I. Sympathomimetics

– noradrenaline

– adrenaline

- isoprenaline (DPE)
- isoproterenol
- salbutamol

II. Adrenergic neuron blocking agents
- guanethidine
- protryptiline
- 6-hydroxydopamine

III. β-receptor blocking agents
- propanolol
- atenolol
- timolol maleate.

Adrenaline is a direct sympathomimetic agent and has both α- and β-adrenergic properties. The α-effect is stimulatory and causes vasoconstriction in the anterior part of the eye, dilation of the pupil and increased outflow. The β-adrenergic effect is inhibitory, leading to inhibition of aqeous humor formation and possibly to an increase in outflow facility mediated by cyclic AMP (18).

Table 1. The fall in IOP after topical adrenaline, as reported by several investigators during glaucoma treatment.

L.-EPINEPHRINE	2%	–8.5 mm Hg (26)
D-EPINEPHRINE	2%	–2.5 mm Hg (26)
L.-EPINEPHRINE	2%	–13.5 mm Hg (6)
EPINEPHRINE	1%	–6.3 mm Hg (19)
EPINEPHRINE	0.5%	–5.0 mm Hg (8)
EPINEPHRINE	0.5%	–3.9 mm Hg (19)
EPINEPHRINE	0.25%	–0.9 mm Hg (19)
		(NOT SIGNIFICANT)

After initial failure, adrenaline was reintroduced by Weekers (25, 26) to manage open angle glaucoma. Table 1 shows the intraocular pressure (IOP) decreasing effect of adrenaline as reported by several investigators during glaucoma treatment. After topical adrenaline there is initial inhibition of aqueous humor production (7) overlapped by an increase in outflow facility. After treatment for a longer period a further increase in outflow facility is reported (2, 3, 4, 6). Harris (8), in patients with primary open angle glaucoma (POAG), and Obstbaum (19), in patients with suspected glaucoma, reported an increase in outflow facility only when 1% adrenaline or higher concentrations were used. In concentrations below 1% the fall in IOP was due only to inhibition of aqueous humor formation. Recently, Townsend and Brubaker (23) found not only a 38% increase in outflow facility, but also a paradoxical 18.6% increase in aqueous production in normal subjects after 1% adrenaline.

The side-effects of adrenaline are:

ocular – browache, hyperaemia, mydriasis, adrenochrome deposits, superficial keratitis, epiphora, allergic reactions and cystoid maculopathy (aphacic eye).

systemic – tachycardia, hypertension, cardiac, restlessness, fear, tremor, fainting, nausea and anxiety.

The side-effects of a drug can be reduced by lowering either the concentration or the frequency of application. It is also possible to alter the structure of an active agent in such a way that the penetration is improved and less substance of the drug is needed. Due to its hydrophilic and lipophilic properties, dipivalylepinephrine (DPE) penetrates the cornea 100 × more readily than adrenaline. DPE is hydrolyzed to adrenaline by esterases in the cornea during transport and exerts its effect on inflow, outflow and pupil in the form of adrenaline. DPE should not be given in combination with choline esterase inhibitors (1).

Table 2 shows the results of comparative studies on glaucoma patients. The intraocular effect of 0.1% DPE is the same as with 2% adrenaline, but the systemic and extra-ocular side effects are less with DPE (14, 15, 16).

Table 2. Results of comparative studies on glaucoma patients with topical adrenaline versus dipivalylepinephrine.

EPINEPHRINE	1%	–4.8 mm Hg
VERSUS		
DIPIVALYLEPINEPHRINE	0.1%	–4.3 mm Hg
(Double blind one dose study	(16)	
EPINEPHRINE	2%	–21%
VERSUS		
DIPIVALYLEPINEPHRINE	0.1%	–18.6%
(3 M. period, doubled masked study (14)		
EPINEPHRINE	2%	–27.4%
VERSUS		
DIPIVALYLEPINEPHRINE	0.1%	–23.7%
(6 M. period, double masked cross over study (15)		

If the effector cell is potentiated or made supersensitive to adrenaline, then the necessary adrenaline concentration also can be reduced. By denervation, the adrenergic effector cell is made supersensitive to catecholamines. Pharmacological denervation can be accomplished with guanethidine or 6-hydroxydopamine. However, 6-hydroxydopamine results in a true degeneration of the sympathetic nerve endings (24) while guanethidine brings about depletion of the adrenaline stored in the granulated vesicles (5, 22). Both effects are reversible. Guanethidine is believed to increase membrane permeability, leading to release of stored noradrenaline. Re-uptake, normally 90% of the released noradrenaline, is blocked, resulting in depletion. Supersensitivity to catecholamines develops at the effector site (17). The Patersons (20, 21) treated ocular hypertensives with 1–5% guanethidine alone. After an initial fall, the IOP nearly reached pretreatment values after 1 month of treatment. However, adding topical 1% adrenaline produced a fall in IOP of 15 mm Hg which increased the longer treatment lasted. Possible side effects of the combination of guanethidine and adrenaline are: burning, browache, headache, cosmetic objections (red eyes), reading problems, hypermetropization, epiphora, ptosis, hyperaemia, mydriasis, adrenochrom deposits, superficial keratitis, chemosis, maculopathy (aphacic patients), allergic reactions, and tolerance. Slight hyperaemia, mydriasis, and slight or transient ptosis are most frequently seen. By combining the two drugs in one eyedrop and by lowering their concentrations, unwanted side-effects can be diminished. The main problem with guanethidine and adrenaline has not been to maintain the fall in IOP, but to control the side-effects.

Our work can be divided into three studies:

1. A trial with 3% guanethidine and 0.5% adrenaline in one eyedrop (GA-medium), applied twice daily in 33 glaucoma patients for a period of 7 months (9).

2. A trial with GA-medium applied once daily for 4 months in 12 patients with POAG and in 12 with suspected glaucoma (10).

3. A trial with 1% guanethidine and 0.2% adrenaline in one eyedrop (GA-weak) applied twice daily for 7 months in 31 glaucoma patients (11).

In all three studies IOP daycurves consisting of at least 4 measurements were made during and in the absence of therapy. Unless otherwise indicated, GA was always given after the first measurement at zero time. Supplemental treatment was avoided as much as possible. In 33 glaucoma patients (59 eyes) during seven months on GA-medium twice daily, there was an average decrease in IOP of 10.8 mm Hg or 37.5%. If the eyes are divided according to the mean IOP in the absence of therapy, it can be seen that the fall in IOP during treatment was 45% in eyes with an initial IOP above 27 mm Hg and 30% in eyes with an initial IOP between 21 and 28 mm Hg. 46% of the eyes were well controlled, with all IOP's during treatment below 22 mm Hg. In 74% of the eyes all the IOP's in the daycurves were lower than 22 mm Hg except one, and this was not higher than 25 mm Hg, while in 26% the IOP was not controlled. This last group include five patients who required additional therapy. In one patient there was evidence of tolerance. Fifteen patients showed a slight hyperaemia and five had moderate hyperaemia. Transient or slight ptosis was found in seven patients and moderate ptosis in two. Occasionally transient keratoepitheliopathy was seen. The slight hyperaemia and slight ptosis, were acceptable for most patients. Despite the hyperaemia and slight ptosis, we find GA-medium to be an effective conservative treatment for glaucoma. Younger patients respond well and operations can be delayed. Combination with other treatment is easily possible

Tonographic analysis in 10 patients with POAG during the 7-month trial with GA-medium twice daily, reveals that the 44% fall in IOP was due mainly to a 54% inhibition of aqueous formation and, to a lesser extent, to an increase in outflow facility (from 23% after one and three months of GA to 43% after seven months of GA). In seven glaucoma suspects, the 43% fall in IOP during treatment with GA-medium was due to 46% inhibition of aqueous humor formation and a 64% increase in outflow facility. After one month outflow facility reached normal values and the difference in the increase of outflow facility between the two groups of patients is striking (12).

We conclude that during chemical denervation with GA the mechanisms that mediate the increase in outflow facility and the inhibition of aqueous humor production are both supersensitive to topical 0.5% adrenaline.

During treatment with GA-medium we observed a biphasic IOP response. Three hours after GA, the IOP peaked at 3.5 mm Hg over the hypotensive phase. Tonographic analysis of the 3-hour peak reveals that the biphasic IOP response was due to a 36% increase in aqueous humor production three hours after GA application. This was significant at the 2% level (13).

To reduce the ocular side-effects, we performed a trial with 24 randomized glaucoma patients (46 eyes) treated with GA-medium 1 × daily for four months.

134

After a pretreatment period of one month with GA-medium 2× daily, all patients applied GA only once daily at 5 P.M. Only two patients had additional therapy. The mean fall in IOP in 16 patients who were successfully treated with GA once daily was 8.9 mm Hg or 33%, compared to 9.9 mm Hg or 37% with GA twice daily. The main reason for failure was an initially insufficient decrease in IOP. Only one patient showed tolerance. Once-daily is not successful if the average IOP without treatment is over 31 mm Hg. On the 46 eyes, 89% were controlled with GA twice daily and 65% with GA once daily. Three out of four eyes responded just as well to daily as to twice daily administration. Table 3 shows that the side-effects are clearly less when GA is given once daily. When GA-medium is applied before retiring, the undesirable effects such as dilation of the pupil, transient ptosis and reading problems develop while the patient is asleep and are therefore not troublesome. The patients found once daily administration very convenient.

Table 3. Comparison of the side-effects during treatment of the same patients with GA-medium once daily and twice daily.

	after 7 months of 2 dd GA	after 4 months of 1 dd GA
Drops unpleasant	1	–
Burning sensations	1	–
c. alienum sensations	1	–
Reading problems	4	1
Ptosis { slight or transient	2	–
Hyperaemia { slight	8	4
Hyperaemia { medium	1	–
Kerato epitheliopathy	–	–

Another method to reduce side-effects is to decrease the concentrations of the drugs used. We performed a 7-month trial on 31 glaucoma patients, 58 eyes, with 1% guanethidine and 0.2% adrenaline in one eyedrop, GA-weak, twice daily, in the absence of any other therapy. Figure 1 (closed circles) shows the results in 19 patients who were controlled with GA-weak twice daily. The average decrease of IOP was 8.4 mm Hg or 31%. Figure 1 (open circles) shows the results in 12 patients who were not controlled. In four patients this was due to an initially insufficient decrease of IOP, and in eight patients to tolerance.

Tonographic analysis in 14 patients showed a 32% increase in outflow facility and a 26% inhibition of aqueous humor formation. In 64% of the eyes all IOP's in the daycurve were lower than 22 mm Hg except one, which was not higher than 25 mm Hg. The IOP without medication seems to have no influence on the success of the therapy. The side-effects with GA-weak were less than with GA-medium. In nine patients we saw a slight hyperaemia with the slitlamp, and of these nine, two patients reported the hyperaemia themselves. Two patients had slight ptosis and one moderate. It can be concluded that GA-weak is an effective drug for the management of glaucoma with only a few side-effects. The

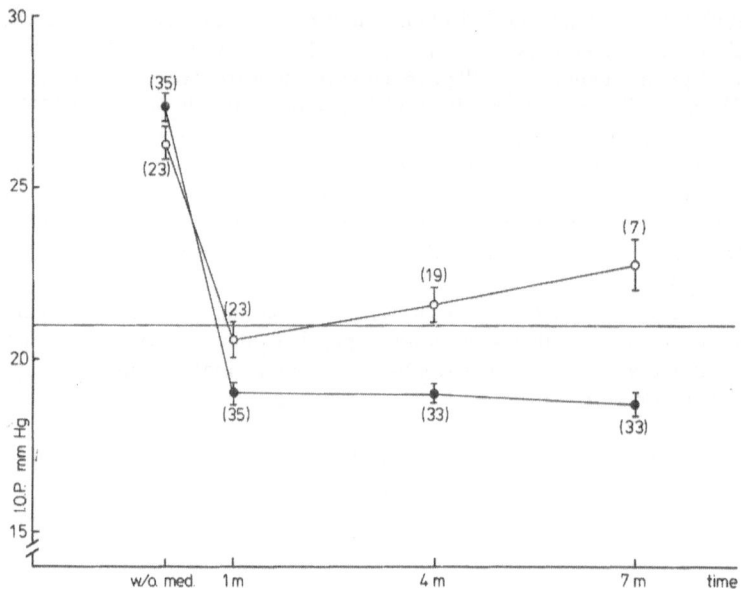

Fig. 1. Mean IOP ± standard error of the mean (SEM) in mm Hg with and without GA-weak twice daily, in 19 glaucoma patients (35 eyes) who were successfully treated (closed circles) and in 12 patients who were not controlled during treatment with GA-weak (open circles).

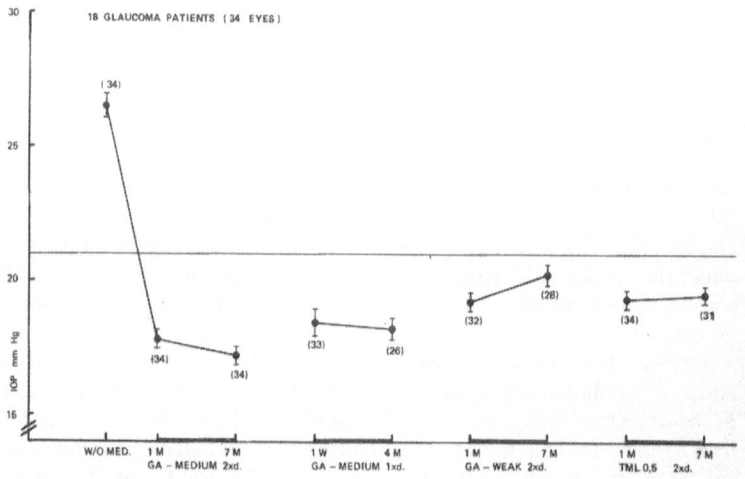

Fig. 2. Mean IOP ± SEM (between bars) in mm Hg in 18 glaucoma patients without treatment and with GA-medium twice daily and once daily, with GA-weak twice daily and with timoptol 0.5% twice daily. All the investigations were performed in the absence of any other therapy.

136

ophthalmologist should be aware, however, that tolerance can develop with GA-weak.

Finally, we compared the results in 18 patients (34 eyes) during treatment treatment with GA-medium twice daily and once daily, with GA-weak twice daily and with 0.5% timoptol twice daily for seven months in the absence of any other therapy (see Figure 2 and Table 4). The mean decrease in IOP in these patients was 35% on GA-medium twice daily, 31% on GA-medium once daily, 24% on GA-weak and 26% on timoptol. With GA-medium twice daily the IOP was controlled (all IOP's in a daycurve less than 22 mm Hg except one but not more than 25 mm Hg) in 94% of the treated eyes, with GA-medium once daily in 71%, with GA-weak in 57% and with timoptol in 65% (see Table 5).

Table 4. Mean fall in IOP of 18 glaucoma patients (34 eyes) during treatment with GA-medium twice daily, and once daily, with GA-weak twice daily and with timoptol 0.5% twice daily, in the absence of any other therapy.

	△ P after 1 month in mm Hg.	△ P after 7 months in mm Hg.	△ P after 1 month in %	△ P after 7 months in %
GA-medium 2 × d	8.7	9.3	33	35
GA-medium 1 × d	8.1	8.3	31	31
	(1 week)	(4 months)	(1 week)	(4 months)
GA-weak 2 × d	7.3	6.3	28	24
TML 0.5% 2 × d	7.2	7.0	27	26

The reasons for failure of the therapy with GA-medium twice daily was tolerance in two eyes; with GA-medium once daily there was an initially insufficient decrease of IOP in eight eyes and tolerance in two. With GA-weak there was an initially insufficient decrease in four eyes and tolerance in ten, and with 0.5% timoptol there was an initially insufficient decrease in three eyes and tolerance in nine. The results in regulating IOP with GA-weak are more or less the same as with timoptol, although the latter has fewer side-effects.

Table 5. Number of eyes controlled in percentages during treatment with GA-medium once and twice daily, GA-weak twice daily amd timoptol 0.5% twice daily. (Number of eyes in parenthesis.)

	GA-medium 2 × d (34)	GA-medium 1 × d (34)	GA-weak 2 × d (32)	TML 0.5% 2 × d (34)
Well controlled	65 (22)	47 (16)	41 (13)	38 (13)
Controlled	29 (10)	24 (8)	16 (5)	27 (9)
Not controlled	6 (2)	29 (10)	43 (14)	35 (12)

In conclusion, the proper way to treat glaucoma patients with GA is as follows.

GA-medium 2 × daily is indicated:

1. If the initial IOP's are very high;
2. If other therapy is unsuccessful;
3. In combination with other therapy to prevent or delay operation.

GA-medium 1× daily is indicated:

1. If the IOP in the absence of therapy is lower than 32 mm Hg;
2. If the patient is uncontrolled with GA-weak;
3. In combination with GA-weak;
4. In combination with other treatments.

GA-weak 2× daily is indicated:

1. If the IOP is elevated, independent of the initial IOP in the absence of therapy;
2. In combination with other treatment;
3. In combination with GA-medium if there is an initially insufficient decrease of IOP or tolerance.

Pharmacological denervation and supersensitivity to adrenaline appears to be very potent combination in the management of glaucoma. However, guanethidine is a highly ionized drug with few lipophilic properties. If it were possible to develop a prodrug of guanethidine with greater lipophilic properties, as has been done with adrenaline, and then combine this with DPE, I think we would have a combination which would lower the IOP very efficiently in low concentrations, with hardly any side-effects.

REFERENCES

1. Abramovski, I. & J. Mindel. Echothiophate prevents hypotensive action of dipivalyl epinephrine. *ARVO abstracts*, p. 165, 1979.
2. Ballantine, E.J. & L.L. Garner. Improvement of the coefficient of outflow in glaucomatous eyes. *Arch. Ophthal.* 66: *314–317* (1961).
3. Becker, B. & A.P. Ley. Epinephrine and acetazolamide. *Amer. J. Ophthal.* 45: *639–643* (1958).
4. Becker, B., T. Petit & A.J. Gay. Topical epinephrine therapy of open angle glaucoma. *Arch. Ophthal.* 66: *219–225* (1961).
5. Csillick, B. Histochemical model experiments on the effect of various drugs on the catecholamine content of adrenergic nerve terminals. *J. Neurochem.* 11: *351* (1964).
6. Garner, L.L., W.W. Johnstone, E.J. Ballantine & M.E. Carroll. Effect of 2% levo-rotary epinephrine on the intraocular pressure of glaucomatous eyes. *Arch. Ophthal.* 62: *230–238* (1959).
7. Goldman, H. Abflussdruck, Minute Volumen und Widerstand der Kamerwassers-tromung des Menschen. *Docum. Ophthal.* 5/6: *278* (1951).
8. Harris, L.S., M.A. Galin & R. Lerner. The influence of low-dose l-epinephrine on aqueous outflow facility. *Ann. Ophthal.* 2/5: *455–458* (1970).
9. Hoyng, Ph.F.J. & C.L. Dake. The combination of guanethidine 3% and adrenaline 0.5% in one eyedrop (GA) in glaucoma treatment. *Brit. J. Ophthal.* 63:*56–62* (1979).
10. Hoyng, Ph.F.J. & C.L. Dake. Maintenance therapy of glaucoma patients with guanethidine 3% and adrenaline 0.5% once daily. In preparation.
11. Hoyng, Ph.F.J. & C.L. Dake. The combination of guanethidine 1% and adrenaline 0.2% in one eyedrop (GA-weak) in glaucoma treatment. In preparation.
12. Hoyng, Ph.F.J. & C.L. Dake. Guanethidine-adrenaline eyedrops in glaucoma

simplex. Production and outflow of the aqueous humor during a long-term treatment. Thesis in preparation.

13. Hoyng, Ph.F.J. & C.L. Dake. Guanethidine-adrenaline eyedrops in glaucoma simplex III. Production and outflow of the aqueous humor during the biphasic response of intraocular pressure. Accepted for publication to *Albrecht von Graefes Arch. klin. Exp. Ophthal.*

14. Kass, M.A., I. Goldberg, A.I. Mandell, & B. Becker. Comparison of dipivefrin and epinephrine in the treatment of elevated intraocular pressure. *ARVO abstracts*, p. 165, 1979.

15. Kohn, A.N., A.P. Moss, N.E. Harget, R. Ritch, H. Smith & H. Podos. Dipivalyl epinephrine and epinephrine. *Amer. J. Ophthal.* 87: *196–201* (1979).

16. Krieglstein, G.K. & W. Leydhecker. The dose-response relationship of dipivalyl epinephrine in open angle glaucoma. *Albr. v. Graefes Arch. f. Klin. Exp. Ophthal.* 205: *141–146* (1978).

17. Mitchell, J.R. & J.A. Oates. Guanethidine and related agents. I. Mechanism of selective blockade of adrenergic neurons and its antagonism by drugs. *J. Pharm. Exp. Ther.* 172: *100–107* (1970).

18. Neufeld, A.H. Influences of cyclic nucleotides on outflow facility in vervet monkey. *Exp. Eye Res.* 27: *387–397* (1978).

19. Obstbaum. S.A., A.E. Kloker. & Ch.D. Phelps. Low-dose epinephrine. Effect on intraocular pressure. *Arch. Ophthal.* 92: *118–120* (1974).

20. Paterson, G.D. & G. Paterson. Drug therapy in glaucoma. *Brit. J. Ophthal.* 56: *288–294* (1972).

21. Paterson, G.D., G. Paterson & S.H.J. Miller. The non-miotic therapy of open angle glaucoma, in Albi International Glaucoma Symposium 1974.

22. Tamura, T. Effect of guanethidine on the vesiculated axon in the dilator muscle area of the rabbit iris. *Jap. J. Ophthal.* 17: *140–146* (1973).

23. Townsend, D.J. & R.F. Brubacker. Acute effect of epinephrine on aqueous formation in the normal human eye. *ARVO abstracts*, p. 164, 1979.

24. Tranzer, J.P. & H. Thoenen. An electron microscopic study of selective, acute degeneration of sympathetic nerve terminals after administrations of 6-hydroxydopamine. *Experientia* 24/2: *155–156* (1968).

25. Weekers, R., E. Pryot, & J. Gustin. Recent advances and future prospects in the medical treatment of ocular hypertension. *Brit. J. Ophthal.* 38: *742* (1954).

26. Weekers, R., Y. Delmarcelle & J. Gustin. Treatment of ocular hypertension by adrenalin and diverse sympathomimitic amines. *Amer. J. Ophthal.* 40: *666–672* (1955).

SUMMARY

The purpose of this study was to evaluate the effectiveness of eyedrops containing guanethidine and adrenaline in glaucoma treatment. The study extended over a period of 4 years and involved 68 patients with either primary open angle glaucoma (POAG) or suspected glaucoma.

The dissertation is divided into two parts: part one contains a pharmacological introduction and part two contains a clinical evaluation of the therapeutic regimen.

Part one

Chapter 1 deals with the anatomy and physiology of the autonomic nerve system with special reference to the human eye and its intraocular pressure (IOP).

Chapter 2 summarizes pharmacological phenomena such as denervation, decentralization and supersensitivity. The effects of denervation and decentralization on intraocular muscles, IOP and aqueous humor dynamics are reviewed.

Chapter 3 and 4 treat the subject of pharmacological denervation. The treatment with guanethidine and 6-hydroxyDopamine with and without adrenaline in experimental animals and in glaucoma patients are surveyed.

Part two

In this part the combination of guanethidine 3% and adrenaline 0.5% as well as guanethidine 1% and adrenaline 0.2% both in one eyedrop in glaucoma treatment are evaluated.

Chapter 6 deals with a double blind short-term trial with guanethidine 3% and adrenaline 0.5% in glaucoma patients. The mean decrease in IOP was 10.1 and 8.7 mm Hg, 6 and 8 h after application respectively.

Chapter 7 contains a seven month treatment of 33 glaucoma patients with the combination mentioned in chapter 1. The average decrease in IOP was 10.8 mm Hg or 37.5%. Patients with an initial mean IOP over 28 mmHg responded with a 44.6% fall in IOP while in patients with an initial mean IOP lower than 28 mm Hg the fall was 30.4%. The IOP was controlled in 74% of the eyes, in which no additional therapy was needed.

Conjunctival hyperaemia and slight or transient ptosis were the most frequent complications. A biphasic pattern of the IOP day curve was observed.

Chapter 8 deals with the verification of the biphasic response of IOP day curve. It was concluded that repeated instillations of guanethidine 3% and adrenaline 0.5% induced a characteristic biphasic pattern in the IOP day curve in patients with POAG as well as in glaucoma suspectes.

Furthermore untreated glaucoma suspects tend to have the highest IOP in the morning while patients with POAG have the highest IOP near noon in daycurves during office hours.

Chapter 9 evaluates the relation between the dilation of the pupil and the course of the IOP day curve after guanethidine 3% and adrenaline 0.5%. It is concluded that the dilation of the pupil has no influence on the course of IOP during treatment.

In *chapter 10* the aqueous humor dynamics during the biphasic response of IOP after guanethidine 3% and adrenaline 0.5% are investigated. During the hypertensive response there is a 36% increase of aqueous humor formation, an unchanged coefficient of outflow and a dilation of the pupil. Hence, it is concluded that fluctuations in the aqueous rate are responsible for the biphasic pattern of the IOP.

Chapter 11 is a tonographic study comparing patients with POAG to glaucoma suspects during a seven months period, with and without guanethidine 3% and adrenaline 0.5%. In patients with POAG the 44% decrease in IOP seems mainly due to inhibition of the aqueous humor formation (54%) and to a less extend to an increase in outflow facility. However, in the patients with suspected glaucoma the 43% fall in IOP was due to an increase of outflow facility (64%) and inhibition of the aqueous humor formation (46%). The increase in outflow during treatment was significantly different between both groups of patients and perhaps the result of degeneration of receptors mediating outflow facility in POAG-patients.

Both groups of patients showed supersensitivity to in- and outflow for adrenaline 0.5%.

Chapter 12 contains a study with a maintenance dose of guanethidine 3% and adrenaline 0.5% once daily over a period of 4 months. The mean fall in IOP was 8.9 mm Hg (33%). Three out of four eyes responded just as well to single daily as to twice daily applications. The advantage of once daily application was a striking decrease in side-effects without markedly affecting the fall in IOP.

Chapter 13 illustrates the combination of guanethidine 1% and adrenaline 0.2% in one eye drop. During 7 months glaucoma patients were treated twice daily with this combination. The average fall in IOP of the patients, who were controlled (64%), was 8.4 mm Hg or 31%. The fall in IOP was due to both inhibition of aqueous inflow (26%) and to increased outflow (32%). There was supersensitivity to in- and outflow for adrenaline 0.2%. It is concluded that lowering of the concentrations of guanethidine and adrenaline resulted in decrease of side-effects and can lead to tolerance.

Chapter 14 contains a review of this study and preliminary results of a comparative study between both combinations of guanethidine and adrenaline in one eye drop and drops of timolol maleate 0.5%. It demonstrates that guanethidine 1% and adrenaline 0.2% lowered IOP and produces equal tolerance compared to timolol 0.5%. However, there were less side-effects with timolol.

In summary both combinations of guanethidine and adrenaline in one eye drop are an enlargement of the therapeutic arsenal of the ophthalmologist in the management of glaucoma. Surgery may be avoided and delayed. However, in view of side-effects a critical approach as to concentration and frequency is required.

SAMENVATTING

Het doel van deze studie is de werkzaamheid en de toepassing van oogdruppels, die guanethidine en adrenaline bevatten, te onderzoeken. Het onderzoek strekt zich uit over een periode van 4 jaar en 68 patiënten met hetzij open hoek glaucoom hetzij oculaire hypertensie namen deel aan de studie.
Het proefschrift valt uiteen in een farmacologische introductie (deel I) en een klinisch onderzoek (deel II).

Deel I

In de farmacologische introductie worden de anatomie en fysiologie van het autonome zenuwstelsel, haar relatie tot het menselijk oog en de oogdruk en farmacologische verschijnselen als denervatie, decentralisatie en supersensitiviteit in het kort behandeld. Het effect op het oog en de oogdruk van guanethidine en 6 hydroxy-Dopamine in combinatie met en zonder adrenaline wordt bij glaucoompatiënten en in experimenten met dieren aan de hand van de literatuur beschouwd.

Deel II

In dit deel wordt de behandeling van glaucoompatiënten met de combinatie van guanethidine 3% en adrenaline 0.5% en van guanethidine 1% en adrenaline 0.2% beide in één oogdruppel geëvalueerd. Na een aanvangstudie, dubbelblind opgezet, waarin de combinatie van guanethidine 3% en adrenaline 0.5% de oogdruk bij glaucoompatiënten 10.1 mm Hg en 8.7 mm Hg, resp. 6 en 8 uur na locale applicatie deed dalen (hoofdstuk 6), werden met deze combinatiedruppel 33 glaucoom patiënten tweemaal daags over een periode van 7 maanden behandeld.
De gemiddelde oogdrukdaling was 10.8 mm Hg of 37.5% . Bij patiënten, die in de aanvang hogere oogdrukken hadden, was de oogdrukdaling percentueel groter. Tijdens de behandeling was de oogdruk in 74% van de ogen gereguleerd. Hyperaemia van conjunctivae en lichte of voorbijgaande ptosis werden vaak als bijwerking gezien (hoofdstuk 7). Tijdens de behandeling werd een biphasische beloop van de oogdrukdagcurve waargenomen en geverifieerd (hoofdstuk 8). De dilatatie van de pupil in de eerste uren na applicatie van guanethidine 3% en adrenaline 0.5% had geen invloed op het beloop van de oogdrukcurve (hoofdstuk 9). Tijdens de hypertensieve fase van de oogdrukdagcurve bleek er een vermeerdering van de kamerwater

145

produktie met 36%, een onveranderde uitstroomcapaciteit en een dilatatie van de pupil in vergelijking met de hypotensieve fase. Dit leidde tot de conclusie dat schommelingen in de aanmaak van het kamerwater de oorzaak zijn van het biphasisch beloop van de oogdrukdagcurve (hoofdstuk 10). Gedurende de periode van 7 maanden, waarin de patiënten met guanethidine 3% en adrenaline 0.5% behandeld werden, werd een vergelijkend tonographisch onderzoek uitgevoerd. De oogdruk daling (44%) werd in de 10 patiënten met open hoek glaucoom veroorzaakt door een remming van de kamerwaterproduktie van 54% en in mindere mate door toename van de uitstroomcapaciteit. Bij 7 patiënten met oculaire hypertensie werd de oogdrukdaling (43%) veroorzaakt door remming van de kamerwaterproduktie (46%) en de toename van de uitstroomcapaciteit (64%). De mate van toename van de uitstroomcapaciteit was significant verschillend tussen beide groepen patiënten en mogelijk het resultaat van degeneratie van sympathische receptoren, die de uitstroomcapaciteit beïnvloeden bij de patiënten met open hoek glaucoom. In beide groepen patiënten was er supersensitiviteit van de mechanismen, die de inhibitie van de kamerwaterproduktie en die toename van uitstroomcapaciteit regelen voor adrenaline 0.5% (hoofdstuk 11).

Vierentwintig glaucoom patiënten werden gedurende 4 maanden met een onderhoudsdosering van guanethidine 3% en adrenaline 0.5% eenmaal daags behandeld. De gemiddelde oogdrukdaling was 8.9 mm Hg (33%). Drie van de vier ogen reageerden even goed op eenmaal daags als op tweemaal daags applicatie. Het voordeel van eenmaal daags appliceren is een opmerkelijke daling van de bijwerkingen met behoud van de beoogde oogdrukdaling (hoofdstuk 12).

Gedurende 7 maanden werden 31 glaucoom patiënten tweemaal daags behandeld met guanethidine 1% en adrenaline 0.2% in één oogdruppel. Bij de patiënten, waarin de oogdruk gereguleerd was (64%), was de oogdrukdaling 8.4 mm Hg of 31%. De oogdrukdaling werd veroorzaakt door een remming van de kamerwaterproduktie met 26% en een toename van de uitstroomcapaciteit met 32%. Zowel de mechanismen, die kamerwaterproduktie remmen, als die welke de uitstroomcapaciteit doen toenemen, waren supersensitief voor adrenaline 0.2%.

Verlaging van de concentratie van guanethidine en adrenaline doet de bijwerkingen sterk verminderen, maar kan tot tolerantie leiden (hoofdstuk 13). Het proefschrift besluit met een beschouwing van de resultaten van bovengenoemde onderzoekingen en geeft een vergelijking tussen beide combinatiedruppels en met timolol maleaat 0.5%.

Guanethidine 1% en adrenaline 0.2% verlaagt de oogdruk in gelijke mate en kan tot dezelfde graad van tolerantie leiden, als timolol 0.5% dat doet, echter met de laatste druppel zijn er minder bijwerkingen (hoofdstuk 14). Samenvattend kan gezegd worden dat beide combinatiedruppels een aanwinst zijn voor het therapeutisch arsenaal van de oogarts in de behandeling van glaucoom. Chirurgie kan uitgesteld of vermeden worden. Met het oog op bijwerkingen die kunnen optreden, is een kritische benadering betreffende concentratie en frequentie van toediening noodzakelijk.

ACKNOWLEDGEMENTS

We gratefully acknowledge the cooperation and the patience of the patients, who made this work possible. We would like to thank Professor C.L. Dake for his help and wise advice, Dr. G.W.H.M van Alphen for his critical comments, Professor R.A. Crone for his editorial advice, Dr. E.L. Greve for reviewing chapter VIII, and Dr. H.C. Innemee for reviewing part one. Furthermore, the help of Mrs. J. Loeb, who performed tonometry, Mr. A. Blijleve, who made the drawings and the help of Mrs. K. Vroom, Mrs. I. Ompi, Mrs. E. Mutsaerts, Mrs. J. Sweers and Mrs. G. Raateland for their administrative assistance is greatly appreciated.

We wish to thank Dr. R.R. Blanken for translation of the manuscript.

We thank Dispersa for providing us with Suprexon 3-0.5 and 1-0.2 during the trial.

Furthermore, we gratefully acknowledge Albrecht von Graefes Archiv für klinische und experimentele Ophthalmologie and Springer-Verlag for their permission to use:
- Graefes Arch. Ophthalm. *203*: 73- 80 (1977) as Chapter VI,
- Graefes Arch. Ophthalm. *214*: 263-268 (1980) as Chapter X,
- Graefes Arch. Ophthalm. *241*: 269-275 (1980) as Chapter XII,

The British Journal of Ophthalmology and the British Medical Association for their permission to use:
- Br. J. Ophthalm. *63*: 56-62 (1979) as Chapter VII.

We wish to thank Documenta Ophthalmologica for their permission to use:
- Doc. Ophthalm. *49*: 369-377 (1980) as Chapter XI,
- Doc. Ophthalm. *49*: 379-388 (1980) as Chapter XIII,
- Doc. Ophthalm. Proc. Series, *22*: 303-311 (1979) as Chapter XIV and Chapters VIII and IX (Doc. Ophthalm., in press).

We thank:
- Dr. A. Moses and the C.V. Mosby Company for their permission to use Figure 1 (Adler's: Physiology of the eye, page 328, 1975),
- Dr. G.W.H.M. van Alphen and the Investigative Ophthalmology and Visual Science for their permission for Figure 6 (Invest. Ophthalm. *15*: 502 Table 2, 1976);
- Dr. F. J. Macri and S.J. Cevario for their permission for Figure 7 from 'The Formation and Inhibition of aqueous humor production. A proposed mechanism of action'. Arch. Ophthalm. *96*: 1664 (1978) Copyright 1978 American Medical Association;

– Dr. G.D. Paterson and Dr. G. Paterson and the British Medical Association for their permission for Figures 9 and 10 from 'Drug therapy of glaucoma'. Brit. J. Ophthalm. *56*: 288 (1972); and

– Drs. D.E.P. Jones, D.A. Norton and D.J.G. Davies; and the Ophthalmological Society of the United Kingdom for their permission for Figure 11 (Trans. Ophthalm. Soc. U.K. *97*: 192, 1977).